Intra-aortic Balloon Pump Therapy

Intra-aortic Balloon Pump Therapy

Edited by
Gerald A. Maccioli, M.D.

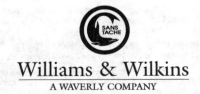

Williams & Wilkins
A WAVERLY COMPANY

BALTIMORE • PHILADELPHIA • LONDON • PARIS • BANGKOK
BUENOS AIRES • HONG KONG • MUNICH • SYDNEY • TOKYO • WROCLAW

Executive Editor: Carroll C. Cann
Managing Editor: Tanya Lazar
Production Coordinator: Peter J. Carley
Book Project Editor: Arlene C. Sheir-Allen
Designer: Cathy Cotter
Illustration Planner: Peter J. Carley, Mario Fernández
Cover Designer: Cathy Cotter
Composition: Mario Fernández
Manufacturing: George H. Buchanan Co.

Library of Congress Cataloging-in-Publication Data

Theory and practice of intra-aortic balloon pump therapy / edited by Gerald A. Maccioli
   p. cm.
  Includes bibliographical references and index.
  ISBN 0-683-05302-7
  1. Intra-aortic balloon counterpulsation. I. Maccioli, Gerald A.
  [DNLM: 1. Intra-Aortic Balloon Pumping. 2. Heart Diseases—therapy. WG 168 T396 1997]
  RC684.I58T48 1997
  617.4'12—dc20
  DNLM/DLC
  for Library of Congress   96-14625
                                                 CIP

Call our customer service department at **(800) 638-0672** for catalog information or fax orders to **(800) 447-8438.** For other book services, including chapter reprints and large quantity sales, ask for the Special Sales Department.

To purchase additional copies of this book, call our customer service department at **(800) 638-0672** or fax orders to **(800) 447-8438.** For other book services, including chapter reprints and large quantity sales, ask for the Special Sales Department.

Canadian customers should call **(800) 268-4178**, or fax **(905) 470-6780.** For all other calls originating outside of the United States, please call **(410) 528-4223** or fax us at **(410) 528-8550.**

Visit Williams & Wilkins on the Internet: http://www.wwilkins.com or contact our customer service department at **custserv@wwilkins.com.** Williams & Wilkins customer service representatives are available from 8:30 am to 6:00 pm, EST, Monday through Friday, for telephone access.

97 98 99 99
1 2 3 4 5 6 7 8 9 10

Dedication

To my wife Sandy, and my children Remy and Allie, for the joy they bring to my life. To my parents, for instilling a deep love of learning.

Foreword

Intra-aortic balloon counterpulsation provides us the unique and potentially life-saving ability to render diastolic augmentation and afterload reduction to the ischemic myocardium. Few technologies bring together the skills of a multidisciplinary team more searchingly. Cardiologist, surgeon, anesthesiologist, perfusionist, and nurse—each has his/her role to play in the application of this device for the care of the patient. In this timely and pertinent textbook, Gerald Maccioli has brought together a distinguished group of contributors from all these areas of expertise.

Gregory Dehmer, Peter Starek, and Edward Norfleet launch the book superbly with an overview of the development of balloon counterpulsation during the last four decades. They weave a fascinating historical web, from the seminal work of the brothers Kantrowitz, through its brilliant application by the engineer Topaz, to the first clinical report of human use by Adrian Kantrowitz in 1968. Decade by decade, the chapter authors document the application of balloon counterpulsation in cardiogenic shock, ventricular failure after cardiopulmonary bypass, and in the support of complicated acute myocardial infarction. Then, with the advent of percutaneous insertion, they lead us into contemporary uses such as failed angioplasty and as an adjunct to reperfusion therapy. The perspective is rounded off with descriptions of lesser known or erstwhile applications, such as a bridge to transplantation, pulmonary artery counterpulsation, and septic shock.

Three chapters follow on technical aspects of balloon design and function. Raymond Shedlick and Gerald Maccioli examine the two commonly used balloon inflation gases, carbon dioxide and helium. They weigh the advantage of high blood solubility of carbon dioxide against that of the low viscosity of helium. They conclude that, given the low risk of balloon rupture, helium provides the optimal performance characteristics for the patient sick enough to require balloon counterpulsation. David Tate highlights the important aspects of balloon design, sizing, placement, and insertion. Warner Lucas and Mark Anstadt provide an elegant exposition on triggering and timing of balloon counterpulsation, its integration with the cardiac cycle, and the quest to determine the ideal indices of myocardial oxygen balance. These authors emphasize the importance of initiating inflation at end systole to maximize diastolic augmentation and coronary blood flow, and initiating deflation at a point in diastole that minimizes end-diastolic pressure and facilitates afterload reduction. Useful clinical pointers on trigger signals and lucid pressure and flow graphics round off a chapter that literally goes to the heart of the matter.

Chapter 5 is divided into three sections that elucidate the use of balloon counterpulsation in different clinical situations. Robin Boineau and Brian Annex explore the use of balloon counterpulsation in patients undergoing noncardiac surgery. They remind us that there are well-established predictors of perioperative cardiac ischemic complications that indicate when prophylactic coronary revascularization or percutaneous coronary angioplasty (PTCA) may be appropriate. When these procedures are not an option, and cardiac risk is high, balloon counterpulsation could prevent cardiac ischemic complications. Unfortunately, their recommendation must perforce be based on anecdotal cases, because no controlled studies presently exist.

Robert Applegate, Gregory Braden, and Michael Kutcher provide an in-depth review of the application of balloon counterpulsation in the cardiac catheterization laboratory. They clarify the role of balloon counterpulsation in patients undergoing high-risk angioplasty by presenting an algorithm based on area at risk, ventricular function, and hemodynamic stability. These authors also underline the importance of balloon counterpulsation in reversing ischemic ventricular dysfunction and hemodynamic compromise complicating coronary atherectomy, failed PTCA, or refractory angina. They emphasize the crucial role balloon counterpulsation plays when acute myocardial infarction is complicated by cardiogenic shock. In appropriate cases, the combination of balloon counterpulsation with emergent coronary revascularization, mitral valve replacement, or ventricular septal defect repair can substantially improve outcome. Finally, the authors offer the tantalizing possibility that diastolic augmentation may prevent coronary reocclusion following primary PTCA or thrombolytic therapy in the face of acute myocardial infarction.

Mark Anstadt and Mark Newman describe the application of balloon counterpulsation to postcardiotomy support, which today accounts for 30 to 50% of its overall use. After an excellent review of the principles of ventricular hemodynamics and the benefits of counterpulsation, these authors present a very logical algorithm for the management of postcardiotomy pump failure. Drs. Anstadt and Newman make the telling point that in patients requiring balloon counterpulsation after cardiopulmonary bypass, postoperative mortality remains a forbidding 40%. In contrast, when balloon counterpulsation is started preoperatively, the mortality rate is only 9%. The authors make a plea for prospective controlled studies to develop objective indications for perioperative balloon counterpulsation; currently, these studies do not exist.

Andrea Baldyga gives us a remarkably detailed account of the risk factors and complications of intra-aortic balloon pump (IABP) therapy, which she approaches from a historical perspective. Thus, we read that during the first decade of its use, the incidence of vascular ischemia was 10 to 15%, requiring surgical intervention one half to one third of the time. Although the advent of percutaneous and then wire-guided placement facilitated rapid insertion, the incidence of vascular complications has actually increased–probably because balloons are being forced into more diseased vessels. Dr. Baldyga discusses the insertion of IABP through existing vascular grafts and the thoracic aorta, and provides an erudite discussion on the prevention, early detection, and treatment of vascular complications. The chapter concludes with sections on balloon entrapment, rupture, gas embolism, and complications such as neurologic and splanchnic injury, thrombocytopenia, and infection.

A wonderfully practical chapter on nursing care during balloon counterpulsation is provided by Betty Sadaniantz. It is of value to physicians as well, not only to increase their appreciation of the vital role of the nursing staff in the safe and effective application of balloon counterpulsation, but also because it provides a number of useful clinical insights not covered elsewhere in the book. Ms. Sadaniantz provides us with a detailed description of the IABP setup and insertion procedure, with an emphasis on monitoring and safety issues and the early detection of complications. A similar approach is taken to balloon maintenance, including important issues such as psychological and family support, hemodynamic monitoring, and positioning. We are given a lucid overview of the maintenance of appropriate balloon timing, together with a useful chart on troubleshooting. Finally, there are excellent sections on IABP weaning and removal.

In the last chapter, David Fehr and Karen High provide an important perspective on the role of ventricular assist devices *vis-à-vis* balloon counterpulsation, either in support of postcardiotomy cardiogenic shock or as a bridge to cardiac transplantation. The authors present a short, clear exposition on the Abiomed, Hemopump, Novacor, Pierce-Donachy, and HeartMate devices and the centrifugal pump. It is of particular interest to note that the HeartMate is the first Food and Drug Administration–approved device marketed as a bridge to cardiac transplantation, and that thrombosis is virtually eliminated by the development of a pseudointimal surface layer that reduces the risk of thrombus formation. Last, the authors remind us that the high incidence of bleeding, infection, and thrombosis remains a formidable limitation to the use of ventricular assist devices.

Intra-aortic Balloon Pump Therapy assumes a basic familiarity with the fundamental principles and application of intra-aortic balloon counterpulsation: this book is not for the neophyte. Nonetheless, it is so lucidly written, with such a wealth of illuminating figures, that it is accessible to professionals of any discipline. Dr. Maccioli has demonstrated a particularly deft touch in encouraging his authors to include paragraph-long quotations from classic citations, which lend vivid authenticity to the text. The result is an authoritative textbook that I am confident will remain the nonpareil reference work on balloon counterpulsation well into the next millennium.

Robert N. Sladen, M.B.Ch.B., M.R.C.P.(UK), F.R.C.P.(C)

Preface

Intra-aortic balloon pump therapy (IABP) has a brief but fascinating history in the world of cardiac surgery and critical care medicine. In fact, early models of our modern device may have been just as great a danger to the patient as their disease. Today, we practice on the shoulders of giant visionaries who have made IABP catastrophe uncommon.

Intra-aortic balloon pump therapy crosses several medical specialties: anesthesiology, critical care medicine, cardiology, and cardiothoracic surgery, as well as the nursing profession, and perfusion technology.

The clinical care of patients requiring IABP therapeutic intervention usually involves all of these disciplines; thus, our goal was to produce a multidisciplinary textbook that would involve all of these fields. Like most multiauthored textbooks, some repetition exists between chapters. I have tried to minimize this but retained any cross coverage that enhances each chapter's ability to stand on its own. Medicine is an imperfect science, fact and opinion are often intertwined, and any errors of commission are unintended.

Gerald A. Maccioli

Acknowledgments

The editor thanks Lisa Baylis for her unflagging secretarial assistance, and Tanya Lazar and Carroll Cann of Williams & Wilkins for the opportunity to edit this book.

Contributors

Brian Annex, M.D.
Assistant Professor of
  Medicine/Cardiology
Duke University Medical Center
VA Medical Center
Durham, NC

Mark P. Anstadt, M.D.
Fellow in Cardiothoracic Surgery
Duke University Medical Center
Durham, NC

Robert J. Applegate, M.D.
Associate Professor
Department of Internal
  Medicine/Cardiology
Bowman Gray School of Mecicine
Winston-Salem, NC

Andrea P. Baldyga, M.D.
Former Associate Director Cardiac
  Surgery, Intensive Care Unit
Department of Cardiothoracic
  Surgery
The Cleveland Clinic Foundation
Presently Graduate Divinity Student
Cambridge, MA

Robin E. Boineau, M.D.
Senior Fellow/Cardiology
Duke University Medical Center
Durham, NC

Gregory A. Braden, M.D.
Assistant Professor
Department of Internal
  Medicine/Cardiology
Bowman Gray School of Medicine
Winston-Salem, NC

Gregory J. Dehmer, M.D., F.A.C.C.,
  F.A.C.P.
Associate Professor of Medicine
Director, C.V. Richardson Cardiac
  Catheterization Laboratory
Department of Internal Medicine
University of North Carolina School
  of Medicine
North Carolina Memorial Hospital
Chapel Hill, NC

David M. Fehr, M.D.
Assistant Professor
Department of Anesthesia
Milton S. Hershey Medical Center
Penn State University
Hershey, PA

Kane M. High, M.D.
Associate Professor
Division of Respiratory/Intensive Care
Department of Anesthesiology
Milton S. Hershey Medical Center
Penn State University
Hershey, PA

Michael A. Kutcher, M.D.
Associate Professor
Department of Internal
  Medicine/Cardiology
Bowman Gray School of Medicine
Winston-Salem, NC

Warner J. Lucas, D.D.S., M.D.
Associate Professor of Anesthesiology
Director, Cardiac and Thoracic
  Anesthesia
Department of Anesthesiology
University of North Carolina
Chapel Hill, NC

Gerald A. Maccioli, M.D.
Staff Physician
Anesthesiology/Critical Care Medicine
Raleigh Anesthesia
    Associates/Critical Health
    Systems, Inc.
Raleigh, NC

Mark F. Newman, M.D.
Chief, Division of Cardiac Anethesia
Assistant Professor
Department of Anesthesiology
Duke University Medical Center
Durham, NC

Edward A. Norfleet, M.D.
Professor and Vice-Chairman
Department of Anesthesiology
University of North Carolina
Chapel Hill, NC

Betty T. Sadaniantz, R.N., M.S.N.,
    C.C.R.N.
Clinical Instructor
Department of Nursing
Rhode Island College
Barrington, RI

Raymond R. Shedlick, CRNA
Staff Anesthetist
Raleigh Anesthesia Associates
Raleigh, NC

Peter J. K. Starek, M.D.
Professor
Division of Cardiothoracic Surgery
Department of Surgery
University of North Carolina
Chapel Hill, NC

David A. Tate, M.D.
Assistant Professor of Medicine
Division of Cardiology
Department of Internal Medicine
School of Medicine
University of North Carolina
Chapel Hill, NC

Contents

1

"An investigation was undertaken to determine whether the blood supply through narrowed coronary arteries could be improved by delaying the arterial pressure wave so that it arrives in the coronary arteries during diastole."(1)

ADRIAN KANTROWITZ, MD, and ARTHUR KANTROWITZ, PhD 1953

History of Intra-aortic Balloon Pump Therapy

Gregory J. Dehmer ▪ Peter J. K. Starek
▪ Edward A. Norfleet

Early Experimental and Clinical Studies

In the early 1950s, as experimental cardiopulmonary bypass techniques were being developed, other investigators were interested in devising mechanical methods to aid the failing ventricle or improve coronary blood flow. In 1953, Adrian Kantrowitz, a physician, and his brother, Arthur Kantrowitz, a professor of engineering at Cornell University, published their work entitled "Experimental Augmentation of Coronary Flow by Retardation of the Arterial Pressure Pulse."(1) In the years before their paper was published, there had been numerous surgical attempts to increase the blood supply to ischemic myocardium. These included operations to promote the development of extracoronary collaterals by creating pericardial adhesions or suturing vascular structures like the omentum, muscle flaps, or lung to the surface of the heart.(2-4) Other operations, such as the Vineberg procedure, involved implantation of the internal mammary artery directly into the left ventricular myocardium. This procedure was designed to promote the development of intracoronary collaterals.(5,6) All of these operations had occasional successes but many failures, and thus, these operations were abandoned. The work of Kantrowitz and Kantrowitz was based on two fundamental physiological observations. It had long been known that contraction of the left ventricle provided the pressure force for movement of blood into the coronary arteries. However, it was also known that left ventricular contraction caused compression of the coronary microcirculation which, in turn, provided resistance to coronary flow during systole. Kantrowitz postulated that if one could perfuse the coronary bed with higher pressures during diastole, when intramyocardial resistance is lower, coronary blood flow would increase during the diastolic portion of the cardiac cycle.(1) Moreover, the higher pressure applied during diastole would dilate the coronary arteries to a greater degree and thus, more flow would occur. This novel concept of increasing pressure during diastole would later become known as "counterpulsation." Their experimental canine preparation, shown in Figure 1.1, was relatively simple. The left circumflex coronary artery was cannulated and two external circuits were constructed to perfuse the distal coronary bed. In one circuit, arterial blood was obtained from the aortic arch via a cannula in the brachiocephalic artery and then shunted through rigid tubing to the circumflex artery cannula. In the other circuit, arterial blood, obtained from the femoral artery, was shunted through a long piece of tubing to the circumflex cannula. By altering the length of tubing between the femoral access site and the circumflex cannula, the arrival of the peak of the pressure wave into

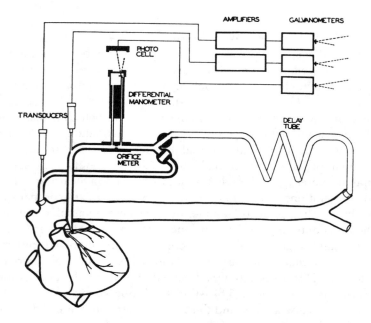

Figure 1.1. *Diagram of the experimental apparatus used by Adrian and Arthur Kantrowitz in their original work on counterpulsation. See text for explanation. (Reprinted with permission from Kantrowitz A, Kantrowitz A. Experimental augmentation of coronary flow by retardation of the arterial pressure pulse. Surgery 1953;34:682.)*

the distal circumflex artery could be delayed until diastole. After optimizing the diameter and length of the external tubing, increases in circumflex blood flow between 22 and 53% were observed. This early experimental model provided the basic physiological concept for counterpulsation as it is applied today.

Approximately 5 years later, Kantrowitz published a second paper using the principle of counterpulsation. This paper, entitled "The Experimental Use of the Diaphragm as an Auxiliary Myocardium," described experiments designed to use the motor power of the diaphragm to share the workload of the myocardium.(7) Two groups of canine experiments were performed. In one group, the mobilized diaphragm was wrapped around the heart and the phrenic nerve was stimulated in systole. Unfortunately, arterial pressure was the only variable monitored, and it was not significantly higher than in the control animals. Although this approach was deemed a failure at the time, there has been recent renewed interest in cardiomyoplasty, a surgical procedure to provide auxiliary muscle to the left ventricle.(8) In the other group of dogs, the mobilized diaphragm was wrapped around the descending thoracic aorta and the phrenic nerve was stimulated in diastole. Both diastolic and mean pressure in the aorta were increased by diaphragmatic counterpulsation, whereas peak systolic pressure was reduced slightly. In this paper, Kantrowitz even questioned the feasibility of constructing an electronic device to regulate contraction of the diaphragm, thus eliminating the need for external electrodes through the skin.

Others adopted the concept of counterpulsation and began to construct devices for clinical applications. One of the first of these devices was the proportioning pump, or arterial counterpulsator, described by Clauss and co-workers in 1961.(9) Clauss wrote:

> *"It appeared likely that if a quantity of blood was withdrawn from the arterial system, at or immediately following the normal instant of isometric contraction, the pressure required in the phase of the maximal rate of ejection would be reduced considerably. If this same quantity of blood was returned during diastole to effect a mean pressure as great as the control pressure, the absolute perfusion would be equal. The coronary artery perfusion relative to the decreased myocardial work would be enhanced."(9)* ROY H. CLAUSS, MD 1961

In the model of Clauss et al, arterial blood was obtained from a major artery during systole and returned by the pump during diastole using the same cannula (Fig. 1.2). When activated in an experimental animal, this device reduced systolic pressure and augmented diastolic pressure. These investigators noted that the ability to induce these pressure changes was dependent on several important variables including the volume of blood displaced, the pressure-volume relationship of the aorta, the position and

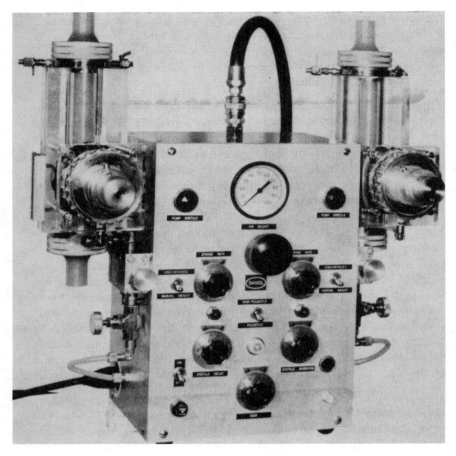

Figure 1.2. *The electronic actuator and ventricles of the arterial counterpulsator developed by Clauss and colleagues.(9) (Reprinted with permission from Clauss RH, Birtwell WC, Albertal G, et al. Assisted circulation. I. The arterial counterpulsator. J Thorac Cardiovasc Surg 1961;42:451.)*

size of the arterial cannula, and proper synchronization with the cardiac cycle. This device achieved the desired physiological results; however, the physical movement of blood occurred relatively slowly and caused too much trauma to formed elements of the blood to be clinically useful.(10) Other investigators, including Harken, Lefemine, Deterling, Birtwell and Soroff, tried to achieve counterpulsation by withdrawing blood from the femoral artery just before systole and pumping it back into the patients during diastole. (11–13) However, pumping blood in and out of the femoral artery produced a considerable amount of hemolysis, and the augmentation achieved was limited because the viscosity of blood allowed only approximately 10 mL to be pumped during a diastolic period.

In 1961, a significant breakthrough occurred in the research laboratory of Dr. W.J. Kolff at the Cleveland Clinic. A young mechanical engineer, Steven Topaz, had just joined a group of researchers who were working toward building an artificial heart. A major problem confronting these investigators was blood damage at the flow rates necessary for adequate perfusion. Recalling how the idea for an intra-aortic balloon pump was conceived, Topaz later wrote:

> *"The answer to the problem was obvious—not to handle the blood—not to pump it! This suggestion brought a great deal of laughter and some hilarity, along with a few ludicrous suggestions. One was to put a balloon in the animal. This idea seemed to be on the same level with the other proposals, except that someone observed that we could pump air very fast without handling blood. The driving equipment was already available and attached. Another solenoid was connected to the timer and air line. And indeed, the blood flow, simulated by water, was increased 30% in the mock circulation when the balloon assisted. In fact, without the artificial heart working, and with just a good aortic valve, the balloon on its own timer could pump 2 liters a minute by itself (correctly timed for filling and correctly regulated for air flow). The duration of the experiment from the expression of the "absurd idea" to connecting it to a working mock circulation, and testing, had taken 2-1/2 hours."(14)*
>
> STEVEN R. TOPAZ, BS 1978

Dr. Spyridon Moulopoulos, a cardiologist working in the laboratory, provided the clinical link for many of these ideas. The first balloon pump described previously was constructed by tying a 20-cm length of Penrose latex surgical drainage tubing around the end of a polyethylene catheter that contained multiple side holes.(15) The distal end of the tubing was occluded so that the balloon device was inflated and deflated through the side holes. Although far from perfect, this initial effort proved to be remarkably successful in a mock circulatory apparatus. In subsequent experiments, this makeshift balloon was replaced with one made in their laboratory from polyurethane. Air was used as the driving gas in the initial trial, but carbon dioxide was eventually substituted because of its marked solubility in blood should the balloon ever rupture. Animal experiments followed quickly and, as in the mock circulation, balloon pumping increased diastolic pressure and decreased systolic pressure. Nevertheless, an important practical problem remained. Within the hospital, it was easy to provide a source of compressed gas for inflation of the balloon, but there was no powerful vacuum, such as the one that existed in the research laboratory, for the rapid deflation of the balloon. Small portable vacuum pumps were available but could not produce the negative pressure required. In describing how the balloon pump was conceived, Topaz later wrote:

"Then, the second solution occurred to me: to use one balloon to drive the air into the second balloon, but to make the drive balloon so stiff and strong that its springiness would evacuate the balloon in the aorta. This device actually worked better than our wall vacuum system."(14)   STEVEN R. TOPAZ, BS 1977

Not only did this dual-balloon concept solve the vacuum problem, but it also provided a safety control for the gas to insure that the intra-aortic balloon could never be overinflated or leak a large amount of gas. A diagram of this initial balloon apparatus is shown in Figure 1.3. Their balloon pump was tested in the mock circulatory apparatus in the laboratory, in canine cadavers and in live anesthetized dogs. In these trials, Moulopoulous et al made critical observations regarding the timing of balloon inflation and were the first to use the dicrotic notch of the arterial wave form to trigger balloon inflation.(15) When the inflation-deflation cycle was properly timed, their balloon pump had the desired phys-

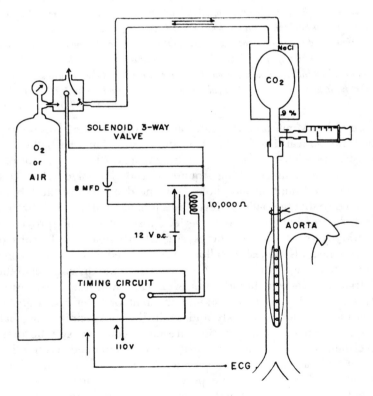

Figure 1.3. *Diagram of the initial laboratory apparatus used by Moulopoulos and colleagues to test the first intra-aortic balloon pump. (Reprinted with permission from Moulopoulos SD, Topaz S, Kolff WJ. Diastolic balloon pumping [with carbon dioxide] in the aorta: A mechanical assistance to the failing circulation. Am Heart J 1962;63:670.)*

iologic effect of both increasing blood flow in the arterial system during diastole and lowering the end-diastolic arterial pressure. The advantages of this approach were obvious compared with earlier devices because blood was not handled outside the body or necessary to prime the device, and only one vessel needed to be cannulated. By the summer of 1961, Dr. Kolff announced to the members of the Cleveland Clinic staff that they were ready to start patient testing. In late September, Dr. Mason Sones, head of the Cardiology and Cineradiography Departments, called asking for emergency assistance with a patient who arrested in the cardiac catheterization laboratory. Within 20 minutes of the call, an intra-aortic balloon pump had been placed in a heroic effort to save the patient's life.(14,15) Although the patient had expired, valuable information was obtained as contrast was injected into the aorta and dye flow into the coronaries was documented during balloon pumping. These ideas and innovations provided the cornerstones upon which modern counterpulsation therapy has been built.

Kantrowitz expanded the initial work from the Cleveland Clinic, conducting several experimental studies in his own laboratory that led to further improvements. He developed a nonocclusive polyurethane balloon and substituted helium for carbon dioxide to expand the balloon.(16) Helium was used because it was twenty times less dense than carbon dioxide and could be shuttled back and forth much quicker through smaller tubes. In January 1968, Kantrowitz and associates reported the first clinical use of intra-aortic balloon pumping.(17)

> *"Our intra-aortic cardiac assistance system for patients in cardiogenic shock following myocardial infarction consists of a catheter and balloon inserted through a femoral arteriotomy into the thoracic aorta. The pumping chamber, activated by helium, is synchronized with the heart by signals from the electrocardiogram or the central aortic pressure transducer."(17)*   ADRIAN KANTROWITZ 1968

The balloon catheter used in these initial patients was 4 mm in diameter, expanded to 18 mm when inflated, displaced approximately 32 mL of blood, and was constructed of polytetrafluoroethylene. The first patient treated with this pump was a 45-year-old woman with juvenile diabetes who had had angina for 5 years. She presented with an acute posterior infarction and rapidly developed congestive heart failure and cardiogenic shock. Despite maximum drug therapy typical of this period, her condition deteriorated and a balloon pump was inserted by direct femoral arteriotomy. Before the onset of balloon pumping, all vasopressor medications were stopped. Balloon pumping was used intermittently during a 7-hour period, during which her clinical condition improved with each period of counterpulsation. The pump was removed, and this patient eventually recovered and was discharged from the hospital. The other two patients in this initial report had acute myocardial infarction and cardiogenic shock, but the outcome was not as fortunate. Balloon pumping was successfully initiated in the second patient, with an improvement in hemodynamic status, but ventricular fibrillation occurred, and the patient could not be revived when the pumping was briefly stopped to reposition the balloon. In the third patient, balloon placement was attempted, but was prevented by peripheral vascular disease, and the patient died from cardiogenic shock.

By December 1968, Kantrowitz and colleagues published an expanded clinical series describing the first 16 patients treated with balloon counterpulsation.(18) All of the patients had cardiogenic shock resulting from a recent myocardial infarction, and balloon pumping successfully reversed the shock in all patients. In this series, 13 of the 16 patients recovered from cardiogenic shock, and 44% were long-term survivors (1–11 months). Although the mortality was high, this represented a substantial improvement over the 85 to 95% mortality from cardiogenic shock typical of this decade.(19) Based on these initial encouraging results, widespread interest developed in the clinical application of intra-aortic balloon pumping, and several other investigators began to use this technique. Shortly thereafter, a National Institutes of Health–sponsored cooperative study was organized to study intra-aortic balloon pump therapy in cardiogenic shock. Commercial developers became interested in this new technology and developed systems of their own, with many further improvements during the ensuing years (Fig. 1.4).

In 1969, Summers et al reported their experience using intra-aortic balloon counterpulsation in three patients with acute myocardial infarction and cardiogenic shock.(20) Although all of their patients died from their infarctions, this study was the first to provide comprehensive hemodynamic and arteriographic data in patients during the period of pump support. Mean systolic arterial pressure decreased 8%, mean diastolic arterial pressure increased 21%, and left ventricular end-diastolic pressure decreased by 50% during counterpulsation. Cardiac output during pumping increased an average of 32%, and coronary metabolism, assessed by lactate levels in coronary sinus blood, converted from anaerobic during shock to aerobic during pump support. Summers also showed the feasibility of performing angiography to define left ventricular function and coronary anatomy during balloon counterpulsation. None of these patients suffered from hemodynamic deterioration during angiography, and this observation led to many more studies during the clinical development of intra-aortic balloon pumping.

Bregman et al (21, 22) and Buckley and associates (23) presented further evidence in the early 1970s that balloon counterpulsation could improve or abolish the clinical shock state following acute myocardial infarction. Although each group used a different type of balloon system, the hemo-

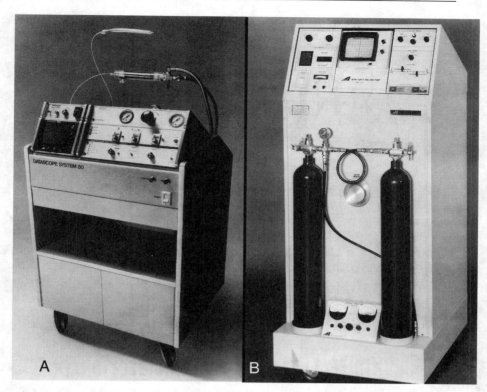

Figure 1.4. *Photographs of the first balloon pump consoles made commercially for clinical use.* **A** *shows the Datascope System 80, which was introduced in 1971, and* **B** *shows the AVCO System 7, which was introduced in 1969. (Photographs courtesy of the Datascope Corp, Fairfield, NJ, and Arrow-Kontron Instruments, Reading, Penn, respectively.)*

dynamic effects and clinical response appeared similar. Bregman used a dual-chambered polyurethane balloon manufactured by the Datascope Corporation (Fig. 1.5). This balloon had a spherical distal chamber that was inflated early in diastole, before the more proximal cylindrical balloon. The distal balloon occluded the aorta, and thus when the proximal balloon inflated, all of the blood was displaced toward the aortic root. In the succeeding systole, both chambers were completely deflated by an active vacuum. Experimental studies showed that this dual-chambered, or unidirectional, balloon caused a 20% greater decrease in left ventricular work and tension-time index and a 66 to 100% greater increase in coronary sinus blood flow compared with a single-chambered omnidirectional balloon. Buckley et al used a triple-segmented balloon developed at the AVCO Everett Research Laboratory. This balloon was designed to inflate from the central segment toward each end. In their series of eight patients, cardiac output increased an average of 400

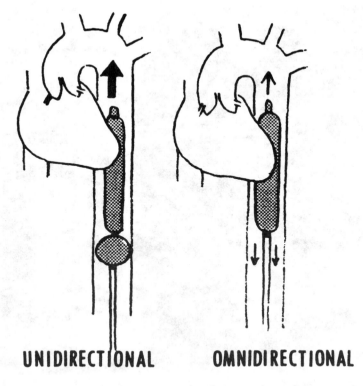

UNIDIRECTIONAL   OMNIDIRECTIONAL

Figure 1.5. *Diagram of the unidirectional versus omnidirectional balloon pump. With the unidirectional pump, the distal round balloon was inflated slightly before the cylindrical balloon. This occluded the aorta distally so that the majority of the pressure generated by inflation of the proximal balloon was transmitted to the coronary and great vessels. Both balloons were deflated during systole. (Reprinted with permission from Bregman D, Kripke DC, Goetz RH. The effect of synchronous unidirectional intra-aortic balloon pumping on hemodynamics and coronary blood flow in cardiogenic shock. Trans Am Soc Artif Organs 1970;16:442.)*

mL/min (3–16%), with a reduction in systolic pressure averaging 9.5 mm Hg and no change in mean arterial pressure.

External Counterpulsation and Other Devices

The idea of external counterpulsation was first described by Dennis in 1963 as a method that was less invasive.(24) Counterpulsation was achieved by encasing the hind quarters of a dog in a pneumatic sleeve. The sleeve was inflated during diastole to compress the arterial bed of the lower extremities and then deflated during systole. Even using this fairly crude device, these investigators were able to demonstrate a reduction in tension-time index and left ventricular end-diastolic pressure while achieving a peak aortic pressure during diastole that was equivalent to the pressure during systole. Soroff et al developed an external counterpulsation device applicable to man and reported the hemodynamic effects in five normal volunteers and clinical results in two patients with cardiogenic shock (Fig. 1.6).(25) In normal subjects, there was a slight decrease in systolic pressure, whereas diastolic pressure increased markedly. One of the two patients with cardiogenic shock showed favorable hemodynamic effects, but both died despite external counterpulsation. The most widely used external counterpulsation device was the Cardiassist–External Counterpulsation System, which consisted of a

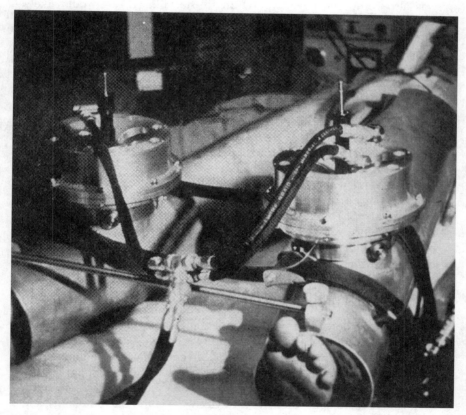

Figure 1.6. *Photograph of a patient in the external counterpulsation system developed by Soroff and colleagues.(25) (Reprinted with permission from Soroff HS, Ruiz U, Birtwell WC, Many M, Giron F, Deterling RA. Assisted circulation by external pressure variation. Israel J Med Sci 1969;5:509.)*

fiberglass leg unit containing water-filled bladders that enclosed the patient's lower extremities. The unit was triggered by the QRS complex of the electrocardiogram and used a hydraulic system to alternately fill or empty the bladders, thereby applying positive or negative pressure to the vascular bed of the lower extremities. The device was simple to use and had the obvious advantage of being completely noninvasive. However, there were several disadvantages of external counterpulsation. First, the movement of water into and out of the leg bladders was much slower than the movement of gas within an intra-aortic balloon. Diastolic augmentation produced by external leg compression was reasonably good, but systolic unloading was less efficient. Systolic unloading is quite dependent on the rapid reduction in impedance at the beginning of left ventricular ejection, and this could not be accomplished by external counterpulsation. Second, since the venous bed of the lower extremities was also compressed, venous return to the failing heart would likely increase, an effect that might be undesirable. Nevertheless, experimental studies demonstrated that external counterpulsation produced several beneficial hemodynamic and metabolic effects. There was a reduction in ST-segment injury pattern and an increase in coronary collateral flow to ischemic myocardial segments, but a variable direct effect on coronary blood flow. (10, 26–28)

Several clinical studies using external counterpulsation were performed. Banas et al (29) reported the relief of stable angina with intermittent external counterpulsation during a period of several days, whereas Loeb and co-workers (30) failed to show that external counterpulsation caused an improvement in myocardial metabolism during angina induced by atrial pacing. Soroff et al treated 20 patients with cardiogenic shock after myocardial infarction and reported five temporary responses, two short-term survivors, and seven long-term survivors.(31) By far, the largest experience with external counterpulsation was the cooperative multicenter trial in which 258 patients with acute myocardial infarction and mild heart failure were randomized to external counterpulsation or standard therapy.(32) The mean duration of external counterpulsation was only 5 hours during the first 24 hours after infarction, and the overall mortality rate between the two groups was not significantly different. However, there was a reduction in hospital mortality in certain subgroups, less recurrent chest pain, a lower incidence of ventricular fibrillation, and an improvement in clinical cardiac functional status at discharge in the group treated with external counterpulsation. Patient discomfort and a feeling of confinement when in the device were common complaints, and there was one fatality due to pulmonary embolism in the treatment group. Questions about the comparability of the patient groups and other statistical issues were raised about this study, and the clinical use of external counterpulsation has never flourished.(10) However, some interest in this technique continues. Lawson and colleagues have reported a short-term improvement in symptoms and thallium perfusion after 36 hours of enhanced external counterpulsation in patients with severe angina and recently published follow-up data showing a sustained benefit in the majority of these individuals after 3 years.(33,34) In these patients, external counterpulsation was postulated to work by facilitating the development, or opening, of coronary collaterals.

Although no other device has achieved the clinical status of the intra-aortic balloon pump, several devices are of historical interest. Two other early counterpulsation devices, tested in only a very few patients, were DeBakey's left atrial-axillary artery bypass pump (35) and Kantrowitz's dynamic aortic patch.(36) DeBakey's device cycled blood from the left atrium to the axillary artery using a pump implanted in the chest and powered by an external gas source. Kantrowitz's dynamic aortic patch was an ellipsoidal silicone rubber pumping chamber implanted in the lateral wall of the descending aorta and powered by an external gas supply. It was inflated during diastole and displaced blood similar to an intra-aortic balloon pump. Both of these devices were abandoned because they required a thoracotomy for implantation and thromboembolic complications were frequent.

The First Decade of Intra-aortic Balloon Pump Therapy (1968–1977)

Intra-aortic balloon pump therapy developed quickly in the 10 years following Dr. Kantrowitz's first clinical cases reported in 1968.(17) During the first decade of intra-aortic balloon pump therapy, all balloon insertions were performed surgically by exposure of the femoral artery and an arteriotomy. Compared with direct insertion of the balloon into the femoral artery, less distal limb ischemia occurred if a short piece of prosthetic vascular graft was sewn end-to-side to the artery so that the balloon could be inserted through the end of the graft (Fig. 1.7).(37) After the balloon was advanced to the proper position in the descending thoracic aorta, the graft was tied off around the catheter, allowing perfusion of the leg to continue, subject only to the impingement of the balloon catheter lying within the femoral artery. Balloon removal was accomplished by surgically exposing the graft, cutting the ligature securing the graft to the balloon, and withdrawing the balloon. Once the balloon was removed, the graft was oversewn and buried in the leg incision and the wound was closed.

Balloons of this decade were fabricated of a flexible, but nondistensible polyurethane membrane, in order to ensure their geometry and volume. The need for rapid inflation and deflation of the balloon dictated the 12 to 14 French diameter of the catheter. (38) During this first decade, intra-aortic balloon insertions were considered moderately complicated, time

Figure 1.7. *Surgical inser-*
tion of an intra-aortic bal-
loon pump using a short seg-
ment of Dacron graft.
(Reprinted with permission
from Wolvek S. The evolu-
tion of the intra-aortic bal-
loon: The Datascope contri-
bution. J Biomater Appl
1989;3:531.)

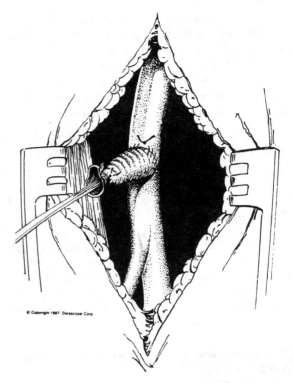

© Copyright 1987 Datascope Corp

consuming, and potentially hazardous; thus, aortic counterpulsation was
often considered as a therapy of last resort. Nevertheless, intra-aortic balloon pump therapy became firmly established as a treatment for cardiogenic shock, and its use expanded to several other clinical situations.
Early clinical experiences that led to some of the established indications
for balloon pump therapy today are outlined in the following text.

Cardiogenic Shock

Based on the initial observations by Kantrowitz and others, considerable
interest developed for the use of intra-aortic balloon pump therapy in
patients with cardiogenic shock after myocardial infarction. During these
early years, the two largest experiences published were the 40 patients
described by Dunkman et al (39) from the Massachusetts General
Hospital and the 87 patients described in a multicenter cooperative clinical trial.(40) The hemodynamic and clinical results were quite similar
between the two studies. Cardiogenic shock was improved or reversed
by intra-aortic balloon pumping in approximately 75% of these patients.
Cardiac output increased 20 to 32% simultaneously with a decrease in
systolic arterial pressure, an increase in diastolic arterial pressure, and a
decrease in pulmonary capillary wedge pressure during balloon pump-

ing. However, the long-term survival rate among those treated with counterpulsation alone was poor: 16% in Dunkman's study and 17% in the
multicenter study. Nevertheless, several key observations that were made
from these studies are still relevant today. First, patients could be catego-
rized into three groups based on their clinical response during the first 24
to 48 hours of counterpulsation. Some patients made such substantial
improvements during balloon pumping that counterpulsation could
eventually be discontinued without a deterioration in hemodynamics or
clinical status. Such patients were felt to have a large component of
reversible myocardial dysfunction causing their initial cardiogenic shock.
A second subgroup of patients failed to have any improvement with
counterpulsation and continued catecholamine support. All died, and
postmortem examinations in some showed large infarctions exceeding
40% of the left ventricle. Finally, the remaining patients responded favorably to counterpulsation but could not be weaned from the device. This
early experience defined the syndrome of balloon dependence, which
still exists today. In both of these early trials, attempts to predict survival,
in advance or from the initial response to balloon pumping, were unsuccessful. Balloon dependence was not a trivial problem, occurring in 64%
of Dunkman's patients and 60% of the patients in the cooperative study.
It is likely that the eventual need to discontinue balloon pump support
and watch a patient lapse into fatal cardiogenic shock stimulated these
clinicians and others to consider coronary bypass surgery in an attempt
to salvage even a few patients who would otherwise die. Once it became
clear that cardiac catheterization and coronary angiography could be
performed safely on patients with balloon pump support,(20, 41) surgery
became the next logical step. With angiographic and operative experience, it became clear that balloon-dependent patients could be subdivid-
ed into those who were balloon dependent because of a large infarction
alone and those who were dependent because of a combination of infarction and reversible ischemia. In Dunkman's report, 40% of those treated
with a combination of intra-aortic balloon pumping and surgery survived. An improvement in outcome with surgery compared with the
poor survival in patients treated with intra-aortic balloon pumping alone
was confirmed in several subsequent uncontrolled clinical trials (Table
1.1).(42–48) Although the management of patients with myocardial
infarction has changed considerably during the past 20 years, intra-aortic
balloon pump therapy remains an important treatment option for the
support of patients with serious left ventricular dysfunction.(49)

Mechanical Complications of Myocardial Infarction

Two uncommon complications of myocardial infarction that can cause
cardiogenic shock are acute mitral regurgitation and ventricular septal
defect. Early in the experience of the investigators at the Massachusetts

Table 1.1

Results of Intra-aortic Balloon Pumping for Cardiogenic Shock
With and Without Surgery

Author: year (reference)	Total number of patients treated	Survival to hospital discharge without surgery (%)	Survival to hospital discharge with surgery (%)
Dunkman et al: 1972 (39)	40	16	40
Scheidt et al: 1973 (40)	87	17	ND
Willerson et al: 1975 (42)	23	5	ND
Baron et al: 1976 (43)	46	28	ND
Hagemeijer et al: 1977 (44)	25	56	ND
McEnany et al: 1978 (45)	145	ND	32[a]
DeWood et al: 1980 (46)	80	48	59
Lorente et al: 1980 (47)	22	17	25
Pierri et al: 1980 (48)	47	8	50

Key: ND = no data.

[a]Most patients in this series treated surgically, but exact number not specified by author.

General Hospital, intra-aortic balloon pump therapy was used to support patients with these events.(50) Counterpulsation resulted in significant clinical and hemodynamic improvement. In those with acute ventricular septal defect, the pulmonic/systemic flow ratio declined in all patients; and in those with mitral regurgitation, the size of the V waves decreased. In the large experience subsequently published by these investigators, cardiogenic shock with acute mitral regurgitation or ventricular septal defect accounted for only 2 and 3%, respectively, of all balloon pump insertions.(45) Although these complications are still uncommon today, intra-aortic balloon pumping remains a valuable treatment when they occur.

Postoperative Pump Failure

During the first 10 years of intra-aortic balloon pump therapy, one of its most important and frequent uses was to support the failing heart in the critical early stages following cardiopulmonary bypass. Typically, this need would arise in patients undergoing coronary or valvular surgery who experienced a "stunned myocardium" following long periods of cardioplegic arrest. Such patients could not be weaned from cardiopulmonary bypass at the conclusion of the surgery or developed profound circulatory failure in the first few hours after leaving the operating room. Many of these patients responded dramatically to intra-aortic balloon pumping. In the early experience at the Massachusetts General Hospital from 1968 through 1976, perioperative assistance was the most frequent reason for intra-aortic balloon pumping, accounting for 30% of all uses.(45) Another large series from the same time period (1965–1979) was reported by the Texas Heart Institute.(51) Intra-aortic balloon pumps were used in 0.03% of 14,168 adults undergoing cardiac surgery with cardiopulmonary bypass. In both of these series, approximately half of the patients responded to the counterpulsation and survived. Table 1.2 summarizes data from several institutions relating to the use of intra-aortic balloon pump therapy following cardiac surgery.(45, 52–61) Although criteria for the placement of an intra-aortic balloon pump in the perioperative period varied among the institutions, its use in this clinical situation was clearly established by these early studies.

During this period, alternative insertion methods were developed to allow for placement of balloon pumps in the operating room, especially in patients with significant aortoiliac disease. The most common of these involved antegrade cannulation of the ascending aorta at the time of sternotomy, either directly or via a prosthetic graft sutured to the ascending aorta.(39, 62–64) The latter method had the advantage of allowing removal of the balloon without a second sternotomy. Today, intra-aortic balloon pumping is still used to support patients in the immediate postoperative period, although less frequently owing to improvements in preoperative medical management, anesthetic practice, and the myocardial protection techniques used during surgery.

Unstable Angina and Refractory Myocardial Ischemia

As experience with intra-aortic balloon pumping increased, its use was expanded to other syndromes of myocardial ischemia. The favorable hemodynamic effects of counterpulsation on the determinants of myocardial oxygen supply and demand led early investigators to consider it as a treatment for myocardial ischemia in the absence of infarction. Two ischemic syndromes felt to require aggressive therapy were recurrent angina in the early phase after myocardial infarction and accelerated angina at rest. It is important to remember that during the early 1970s, therapy for these conditions consisted of bed rest, oxygen, anticoagulation, oral or topical nitroglycerin, and a relatively new drug, propranolol. Intravenous nitroglycerin therapy was approximately 5 years away, calcium channel blockers 8 years away, and the era of interventional coronary procedures for unstable angina approximately 15 years in the future. During this time period, cardiac catheterization in unstable patients was felt to be excessively hazardous. In 1973, the group at the Massachusetts General Hospital published their initial experience with 11 patients, 5 with post-infarction angina and the remainder with recurrent ischemic attacks at rest.(65) The balloon pump eliminated ischemia in nine patients and markedly reduced the frequency in the remaining two. All patients had angiography and subsequent bypass surgery during balloon pump therapy, with a survival rate of 91%. These same investigators pub-

Table 1.2

Early Results of Intra-aortic Balloon Pump Support for Postoperative Cardiac Failure

Institution (reference)	Years of Study	No. of Patients Receiving IABPs	% of Total Surgeries	Survival to Discharge (%)	Time Range of IABP Support
Massachusetts General Hospital (45)	1971–1976	225	$\cong 4$	54	NS
Texas Heart Institute (52)	1972–1979	419	0.03	45	3–195 h
Emory University (53)	1976–1978	62	2.7	65	1–18 d
Yale University (54)	NS	80	ND	36	NS
Columbia-Presbyterian (55)	1972–1974	47	ND	66	Mean = 60 h
University of Miami (56)	1972–1974	43	$\cong 8.6$	58	12–96 h
Loyola University (57)	1973–1975	40	7.1	55	1h–11d
University of Rochester (58)	NS	23	ND	61	2h–13d
Northern General Hospital, Sheffield, England, UK	NS	21	ND	52	1–100h
Boston City Hospital (60)	NS	14	ND	43	2–172h
Peter Bent Brigham Hospital (61)	1971–1973	12	4	58	6–204h

Key: NS = not stated; ND = no data.

[a]Most patients in this series treated surgically, but exact number not specified by author.

lished an expanded clinical experience in 93 patients 5 years later.(66) Sixty patients had unstable angina without infarction, and the remainder had post-infarction angina. Intra-aortic balloon pump therapy eliminated the attacks of ischemia in 81% of the patients and reduced the frequency of attacks in the remainder. All patients were found to have coronary anatomy amenable to surgery, and the overall mortality from revascularization was 5.4%, with a higher mortality (9.1%) in those with post-infarction angina. Perioperative infarction occurred in 2.2%, and survival at an average of 38 months was 95.5%, with 93% of the survivors experiencing no significant angina. Clinical studies from other investigators during this same time period showed similar results.(67, 68) Although intra-aortic balloon pumping is still necessary occasionally to control refractory ischemia, other therapies have markedly reduced the need for counterpulsation in this setting.

Limitation of Ischemic Injury in Acute Myocardial Infarction

During the early to mid-1970s, there was considerable interest in methods to limit the amount of necrosis occurring with acute myocardial infarction. Early experimental data from Maroko and associates suggested that balloon counterpulsation may limit ischemic injury.(69) Using the technique of epicardial ST-segment mapping, the effects of acute coronary occlusion were studied in a canine model of infarction. Even when balloon pumping was started 3 hours after occlusion, the extent and magnitude of ST-segment elevation was decreased. In a preliminary fashion, these investigators also studied two patients in the midst of an infarction with precordial ST-segment mapping before and after the initiation of balloon pump therapy. As in the canine model, an improvement in the amount and extent of ST-segment elevation was observed. Other experimental studies during this time period examined the effects of intra-aortic balloon pumping on coronary perfusion, but with conflicting results. Some investigators attempted to measure changes in regional myocardial blood flow but failed to show conclusively that balloon pumping increased collateral blood flow into an ischemic area.(70–72) However, others showed that adequate counterpulsation could open dormant collateral vessels in dogs.(26, 73) Radiolabeled microspheres were used to directly measure regional coronary blood flow in one study, and flow did increase with counterpulsation.(74) As these and several other clinical studies showed, the effects of counterpulsation on coronary blood flow are complex and dependent on many variables, including the duration of ischemia before balloon pumping, the magnitude of transmural pressure gradient produced by balloon pumping, the diastolic perfusion pressure within the coronary circulation, the presence of collaterals, and the integrity of coronary autoregulation.(75–81) In general, unless the cardiac output was low initially, as in cardiogenic shock, balloon pumping produced little steady-state change in coronary blood flow because of subsequent autoregulation. However, when coronary blood flow was low with the coronary vasculature maximally or near maximally vasodilated due to metabolic factors, balloon pumping produced a large increase in coronary blood flow.

Similar to the variable results of studies that examined the effect of intra-aortic balloon pumping on coronary blood flow, animal studies did not show a consistent reduction in infarct size with counterpulsation.(82, 83) Relatively few clinical studies were performed to evaluate the influence of intra-aortic balloon pumping on infarct size. Based on their large clinical experience with balloon pumping, Leinbach and colleagues at the Massachusetts General Hospital were the first to conduct a clinical trial of this new potential indication for counterpulsation.(84) Eleven patients with anterior myocardial infarction less than 6 hours old and without cardiogenic shock underwent intra-aortic balloon pumping. The patients responded to counterpulsation by either a marked reduction in pain and precordial ST-segment elevation within minutes (n = 5) or a gradual clinical and electrocardiographic improvement not clearly different from the natural history of infarction (n = 6). Hemodynamics before treatment did not predict the response to balloon pumping, but patency of the left anterior descending coronary artery on subsequent angiography did. In all of those who responded rapidly, the artery was patent, whereas it was occluded in five of the six with a slow response. Because there was no control group, it was not possible to determine whether a similar percentage of arteries would have opened spontaneously without counterpulsation. Subsequently, two small randomized trials in patients with acute myocardial infarction failed to find any reduction in infarct size or mortality with balloon counterpulsation.(85, 86) Moreover, emphasis has now shifted to therapies designed to re-establish coronary flow as the means to limit infarct size. Although the available data suggest that intra-aortic balloon pump therapy does not limit infarct size, Leinbach suggested that the counterpulsation may play a role in the maintenance of coronary patency, a concept that has recently received clinical attention.(87)

Serious Refractory Arrhythmias

The concept and application of intra-aortic balloon pump therapy for the control of ventricular irritability unresponsive to pharmacological therapy was first introduced by Mundth and co-workers in 1973.(88) However, relatively few patients have been treated with counterpulsation for this specific indication.(42, 54) In the large experience reported from the Massachusetts General Hospital, refractory arrhythmias accounted for 3% of all balloon pump insertions, and all of these were in the setting of a recent myocardial infarction.(45, 89) Balloon pumping resulted in improvement of the arrhythmia in 86% and resolution of the arrhythmia in 55% of the patients, with an overall survival rate of 55%. In all of these studies, the investigators felt that the ability of balloon counterpulsation to increase cardiac performance and reverse ischemia was the likely mechanism for the alleviation of the arrhythmias. Because the number of antiarrhythmic agents available and their potency have increased, it is now rarely necessary to consider intra-aortic balloon pumping for the relief of refractory arrhythmias.

In summary, the first decade of intra-aortic balloon pump therapy was characterized by initial studies that defined the basic physiologic effects of balloon counterpulsation and numerous subsequent investigations in which the benefits of these physiologic alterations were applied to an expanding list of clinical indications. Some of these indications, such as post-cardiopulmonary bypass pump failure and the support of patients with complicated myocardial infarctions, are still relevant today. Other indications, such as its use in patients with unstable angina or refractory arrhythmias, have been replaced by newer treatment modalities.

The Second Decade of Intra-aortic Balloon Pump Therapy (1978–1987)

Although the value of intra-aortic balloon pumping for several specific indications was established during the first decade of use, the risks of the surgical insertion method were not trivial. Important vascular and local wound complications had been reported in 5 to 36% of treated patients.(90–92) Although not considered a complication as such, attempts to place an intra-aortic balloon failed because of vascular disease or tortuosity in 6 to 29% of patients.(92, 93) The majority of these failures and complications arose because of the need to pass the relatively inflexible, bulky balloon through descending aortas that were often severely diseased. It became clear that an easier method of balloon insertion was necessary to make counterpulsation safer and available to more patients, and this was the major event occurring during the second decade of balloon pump therapy.

Percutaneous Insertions

Methods to allow the percutaneous insertion of balloon pumps were developed separately by the two major manufacturers of balloon pumps during this time period, and their ideas were later combined and adopted by both. In 1978, Wolfson and associates reported their initial experience with a modified AVCO trisegment intra-aortic balloon catheter.(94) Insertion of this balloon was still accomplished by surgical exposure of the femoral artery and the attachment of a small segment of vascular graft; however, the balloon was modified by the addition of a central lumen (1 mm in internal diameter) extending from the tip to a plastic connector near its proximal end. The addition of the central lumen to the standard balloon catheter provided three distinct benefits. First, it enabled placement of the catheter with continuous monitoring of the arterial pressure. Damping of the pressure provided an early clue to the presence of obstruction or intimal dissection. Once the balloon was in position, the central lumen could be used to monitor arterial pressure and to time the augmentation without the need for a separate arterial monitoring line. Second, if resistance was met or damping of the pressure occurred, contrast agent could be injected to document the source of obstruction and possibly get beyond it. Finally, a guidewire, similar to those used for angiographic procedures, could be advanced through the central lumen to direct the balloon around atherosclerotic disease or tortuosity. Wolfson successfully used this balloon in 15 of 16 patients, including 4 of 5 in whom attempts to place a standard balloon catheter had failed, and none of the patients had complications.

At the same time, engineers at the Datascope Corporation were working on different improvements in balloon design.(38) A prototype balloon was developed that allowed one end of the balloon to rotate freely in relation to the other end, which remained fixed to the catheter. This modification allowed the balloon to be twisted on its long axis and wound tightly to reduce its bulk and diameter. Subsequent modifications employed a slender support wire inside the balloon instead of the catheter shaft. This prevented the balloon from coiling upon itself when wound and also provided longitudinal stiffness for advancement into an artery. A miniature bearing was added to the distal end of the balloon, allowing it to untwist spontaneously. As this design was perfected, it was possible to wind the balloon to a diameter smaller than that of the catheter shaft. This allowed the balloon to pass through a 12 French vascular sheath, which could be inserted using the standard Seldinger technique (Fig. 1.8). With this innovation, the era of percutaneous insertions began. The first percutaneous insertion was performed in February 1979, and the experiences with this technique at two centers were published in August 1980.(38, 95, 96) Compared with the traditional surgical method, important vascular complications were much lower (2 to 3%), as was the failure rate for insertions (9.3%). The most striking difference was the speed of insertion, which was less than 5 minutes by the percutaneous route compared with 30 to 45 minutes by the surgical route. A longer vascular sheath was introduced approximately a year later to better deal with iliac disease and tortuosity. With the use of this long sheath, the failure rate for percutaneous balloon insertions was lowered further.(97) Both retrospective and randomized trials comparing the percutaneous method with surgical methods of insertion were subsequently published.(98, 99) Although the percutaneous method was clearly faster and technically easier, the success rate for insertions was similar to the surgical method and major vascular complications were actually increased.

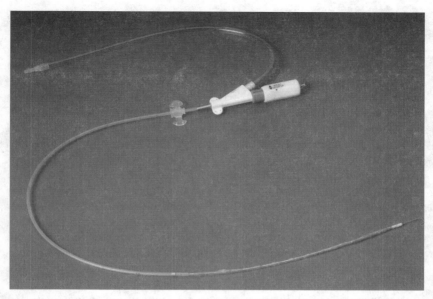

Figure 1.8. *Example of an intra-aortic balloon catheter used during the second decade of counterpulsation therapy. This catheter (PERCOR-DL, Datascope Corp, Fairfield, NJ) was wrapped by turning the white knob at the distal end of the catheter. This diminished the size of the balloon and allowed it to fit through a vascular sheath. A central lumen for a guidewire was also present. (Photograph courtesy of the Datascope Corp.)*

Most investigators felt that the increased complications were, in part, related to the fact that the ease of percutaneous insertion encouraged its use in patients who might otherwise not be considered candidates for balloon pump therapy. Thus, because balloon pumps were being used in greater numbers and in sicker patients, complications were increased. Subsequent research identified diabetes, peripheral vascular disease and female gender as pre-insertion risk factors for the development of limb ischemia. (100)

Improvements in manufacturing and materials technology soon allowed a reduction in catheter diameter from 12 to 10.5 French. By 1985, a pre-folded balloon had been developed that did not require any substantial preparation before placement through the introducer sheath. The only preparation necessary was to use a large syringe to pull a vacuum in the balloon before insertion, thus collapsing it to the smallest possible diameter. This allowed a further reduction in balloon size to 9.0 or 9.5 French if a central lumen was present or 8.5 French without a central lumen.

Expanding Indications for Counterpulsation

Preoperative Use in Patients with Left Main Coronary Artery Disease
During the early development of surgical revascularization of the coronary arteries, it was recognized that patients with critical left main coro-

nary stenosis were at increased anesthetic and operative risk.(53) Because of its favorable effects in supporting the failing heart after bypass, prophylactic preoperative intra-aortic balloon pumping was evaluated as a means to lower risk in this setting. Rajai et al, in a small nonrandomized study, reported no operative deaths when prophylactic intra-aortic balloon pumping was used.(101) However, Vijayanagar and colleagues reviewed the course of 75 patients with greater than 70% left main stenosis who underwent surgical revascularization between 1974 and 1980.(102) In their study population, 85% had unstable angina and 90% had significant right coronary artery disease. Intra-aortic balloon pumps were inserted prophylactically in only four patients preoperatively and were required in two additional patients postoperatively. Balloon pumps were inserted because of medically-refractory angina and not on the basis of coronary anatomy alone. Postoperative myocardial infarction occurred in 4% and death in 2.6%. These data indicated that successful surgical revascularization could be accomplished without the use of intra-aortic balloon pumping. It is likely that improvements in anesthetic and myocardial protection techniques during surgery have diminished the need for counterpulsation as a support mechanism for patients with left main disease. Currently, intra-aortic balloon pumping before surgery for left main disease is more dependent on the clinical presentation, associated disease of the right coronary artery, left ventricular function, and clinical condition after coronary angiography.(103)

Aortic Stenosis
The use of intra-aortic balloon pumping to support the decompensated patient with critical aortic stenosis was reported by Folland and associates in 1985.(104) Patients with critical aortic stenosis were compared with control patients who had unstable angina but no aortic valve disease. There was no decrease in left ventricular systolic pressure, and there was a similar increase in aortic diastolic pressure among the groups. Counterpulsation resulted in a clinically acceptable increase in the transvalvular gradient, a slight increase in stroke volume, and a marked improvement in clinical condition that facilitated successful aortic valve replacement. The improvement in clinical condition was thought to be related to a reduction in coexistent ischemia in these patients.

Use in High-Risk or Failed Coronary Angioplasty
The first focused report of intra-aortic balloon pumping in conjunction with coronary artery angioplasty was in 1983 by Alcan et al,(105) although its use in this circumstance is mentioned in some earlier publications.(98) In the majority of Alcan's patients, the balloon pump was inserted before angioplasty because of clinical instability such as post-infarction angina, unstable angina without infarction, or cardiogenic shock. In the remaining patients, it was inserted for hemodynamic stabi-

lization following early or late vessel closure or before urgent bypass surgery following an unsuccessful angioplasty attempt. Survival to the time of hospital discharge occurred in 93% of these patients. As the application of coronary interventional procedures has evolved over the years, so has the use of intra-aortic balloon counterpulsation support. Although emergency balloon pump therapy is still appropriate in patients with marked clinical instability before or during the procedure, its use has expanded to include hemodynamic support for elective procedures in high-risk patients. Patients considered for such supported angioplasty include: (1) Those undergoing left main angioplasty when the vessel is not protected by patent bypass grafts to the left coronary system, (2) those undergoing dilation of the only remaining conduit to the heart, (3) those with left ventricular ejection fractions ≤ 30% undergoing angioplasty of arteries supplying viable myocardium, and (4) those undergoing multivessel angioplasty complicated by periods of hypotension. In this latter circumstance, intra-aortic balloon pump support may prevent occlusion of previously dilated sites.(106) Four major studies have examined the role of intra-aortic balloon counterpulsation in elective high-risk angioplasty, and the results are summarized in Table 1.3.(107–110) Despite the successful initial outcome in the majority of patients, in-hospital mortality was fairly high (6.2 to 19%) and most likely related to the high-risk clinical and angiographic characteristics among these patients. The exact role of coronary interventions supported by balloon counterpulsation or other techniques remains to be determined in the future.

Bridge to Transplantation

The feasibility of using intra-aortic balloon pump support as a bridge to cardiac transplantation was established during the second decade of balloon pump usage and has subsequently expanded.(111–113) The major effect of intra-aortic balloon pumping in end-stage heart failure is afterload reduction. Intra-aortic balloon pumping represents the ultimate in afterload reduction without resorting to more invasive ventricular assist devices. Although the use of balloon pump support can be lifesaving, the prolonged use of counterpulsation is not without significant complications in such patients. The standard insertion technique through the femoral artery severely limits the patient's mobility and results in confinement in bed. As a result, these already compromised patients are at high risk for the development of pulmonary complications including pneumonia and pulmonary embolism, which may then preclude transplantation. Insertion of an intra-aortic balloon pump through the iliac artery improves mobility and may allow ambulation; however, it requires a retroperitoneal approach for access to the vessels.(114) Insertion techniques via the subclavian or axillary arteries have been reported to allow increased mobility and even ambulation.(115–117)

Table 1.3

Studies of Elective Balloon Pump Support for Coronary Angioplasty

	Anwar et al (107) (1984–1990)	Voudris et al (108) (1987–1988)	Kahn et al (109) (1987–1989)	Aguirre et al (110) (1991–1993)
Total PTCA procedures	8700	1385	3408	1120
% of patients having IABP support	1.1	1.9	0.9	1.9
Mean age (yr)	64	63	66	55
LVEF	≤35%	29±10%	24±8%	35±12%
Multivessel disease (%)	82	100	100	81
High-risk feature (%)				
Poor LVEF	100	89	61	86
Multivessel PTCA	NS	11	NS	NS
Single remaining artery	NS	NS	39	14
Clinical Outcome				
Successful PTCA (%)	86	100	96	95
Myocardial infarction (%)	4.1	0	0	4.7
Emergent CABG (%)	6.2	0	0	0
Procedural death (%)	1.0	0	0	0
In-hospital death (%)	6.2	8	7.1	19
Vascular complications (%)	2.1	8	11	14

Key: PTCA = percutaneous transluminal coronary angioplasty; LVEF = left ventricular ejection fraction; CABG = coronary artery bypass graft; NS = no stated.

Support of the Right Heart

Approximately 2 years after the first clinical use of the intra-aortic balloon pump, investigators began to consider the option of counterpulsation for the failing right heart. Kralios and co-workers constructed an animal model of acute right heart failure by causing pulmonary embolism and showed that intrapulmonary balloon pumping increased cardiac output, decreased pulmonary resistance, decreased right atrial pressure, and increased right ventricular systolic pressure.(118) Subsequent experimental studies confirmed these favorable effects on right heart function, and special balloon shapes tapered to conform to the pulmonary artery were developed.(119–123) The first use in humans of intrapulmonary balloon pumping was reported in 1980 by Miller and colleagues.(123) Their patient was a 53-year-old man with severe coronary artery disease who could not be weaned from cardiopulmonary bypass despite intra-aortic balloon pumping. With each weaning attempt, the right ventricle became acutely distended, and ventricular fibrillation ensued. An intrapulmonary balloon was placed by suturing a Dacron tube graft to the main pulmonary artery, which then served as a reservoir for a standard 35-mL balloon (Fig. 1-9). The patient's status improved steadily during the next 30 hours; however, serious ventricular arrhythmias ultimately led to his death. Although survival after intrapulmonary balloon pumping has been poor, some successes have been reported (124–126).

Transport Capabilities for Balloon Pumping

As technical advances were made in balloon pump catheter design, parallel advances were made in the mechanical and electronic drive consoles used to power the balloon counterpulsation. These innovations led to smaller drive consoles and, eventually, systems designed specifically for transport of critically ill patients (Fig. 1.10). These systems provided this potentially life-saving therapy during inter-hospital transports by ambulance, helicopter or fixed-wing aircraft.(127, 128)

Other Indications

As its benefit in numerous types of cardiac failure was demonstrated, the use of balloon counterpulsation expanded to other clinical situations. During sepsis, there are substantial increases in the demands placed on the heart, which can result in failure or even cardiogenic shock. For patients with septic shock who do not respond to maximum pharmacological support, intra-aortic balloon counterpulsation may increase coronary blood flow, reduce left ventricular workload, and improve tissue perfusion while maintaining an adequate mean arterial pressure.(129,130) Also, intra-aortic balloon pump therapy has been used when cardiogenic shock results from severe blunt trauma to the heart and in the treatment of overdoses of drugs that have powerful negative inotropic actions, such as beta-blockers.(131,132) In such patients, cardiac output is increased,

Figure 1.9. *Schematic drawing of the first use in humans of pulmonary artery counterpulsation. A balloon was placed in the pulmonary artery by first suturing a 20-mm Dacron tubular graft to the main pulmonary artery. The graft functioned as a pumping reservoir for a 35-mL omnidirectional balloon. Note also that a unidirectional balloon was placed in the descending aorta. (Reprinted with permission from Miller DC, Moreno-Cabral RJ, Stinson EB, Shinn JA, Shumway NE Pulmonary artery balloon counterpulsation for acute right ventricular failure. J Thorac Cardiovasc Surg 1980;80:760.)*

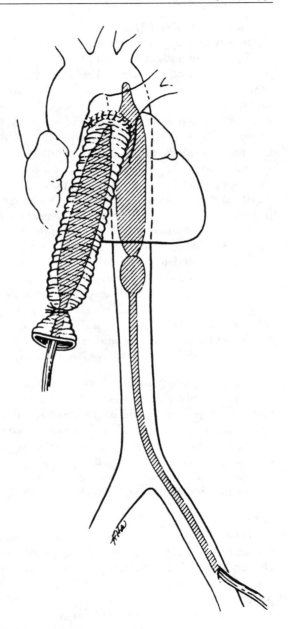

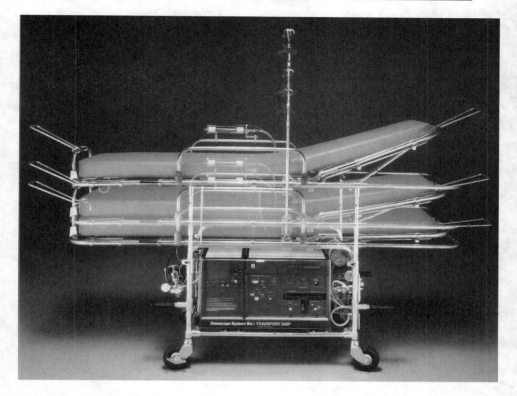

Figure 1.10. *The Datascope System 84A transport pump is displayed with the attached stretcher shown in multiple positions. (Photograph courtesy of the Datascope Corp, Fairfield, NJ.)*

hemodynamic stability is achieved, and peripheral perfusion is maintained until the heart recovers from the insult. Finally, using miniature balloons containing 2.5 to 10 mL of gas, counterpulsation therapy was expanded to infants and children.(133)

In summary, the second decade of intra-aortic balloon pump therapy was characterized by major technical advances in balloon pump design. These led to the percutaneous approach that is now the most common method of insertion. These technical advances allowed balloon pump therapy to be applied to greater numbers of patients, and new indications were explored.

The Third Decade of Intra-aortic Balloon Pump Therapy (1988–Present)

During the last 8 years, additional technical innovations have occurred to enhance the use of intra-aortic balloon counterpulsation as a treatment

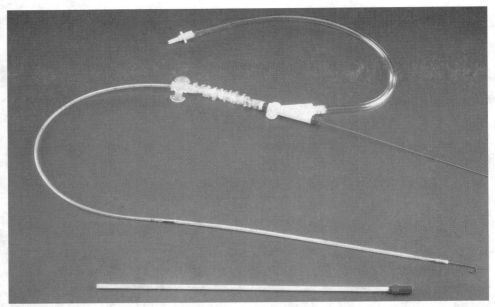

Figure 1.11. *Photograph of a typical intra-aortic balloon catheter (PERCOR STAT-DL , Datascope Corp, Fairfield, NJ) now in use. This catheter can be inserted using the sheath-less technique or with the optional sheath as shown in the bottom of the photograph (Photograph courtesy of the Datascope Corp.)*

modality. The most prominent of these developments has been the modification of the balloon catheter for sheathless insertion.(134) Two changes were made to facilitate the sheathless insertion method. First, the catheter tip was altered from the standard blunt design to a more tapered "ballistic" profile to allow for greater ease of tissue penetration. Second, the proximal end of the balloon was strengthened to fuse the balloon more securely to the shaft and assure enhanced pushability of the catheter without bunching up of redundant balloon material (Fig. 1.11). By eliminating the need for an insertion sheath, the cross-sectional area compromising the femoral artery was reduced from 11.5 mm^2 to 7.0 mm^2 for 9 French and to 7.9 mm^2 for 9.5 French balloons. In uncontrolled trials, use of this technique has allowed rapid and safe insertion, effective counterpulsation and a reduction of limb ischemia from 26 to 9%.(134,135) Other technical advances in electronic and mechanical design have (1) allowed a further reduction in console size, (2) incorporated improved computer algorithms for automated rate and rhythm tracking without user intervention, and (3) provided enhanced diagnostic and alarm systems that display step-by-step troubleshooting procedures and even allow remote monitoring of balloon function by computer modem (Fig. 1.12).

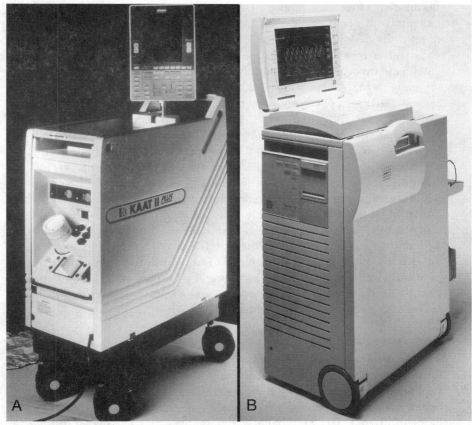

Figure 1.12. *Examples of two balloon pump consoles currently in use.* **A** *shows the Arrow-Kontron KAAT II Plus system, and* **B** *shows the Datascope System 97. (Photographs provided by Arrow-Kontron Instruments, Reading, Penn, and Datascope Corp, Fairfield, NJ, respectively.)*

New Indications for Intra-aortic Balloon Pump Therapy

In several small reports, intra-aortic balloon pumping has been used for high-risk cardiac patients undergoing noncardiac surgery. Grotz and Yeston reported the successful outcome of prophylactic intra-aortic balloon counterpulsation in three patients with coronary artery disease and impaired left ventricular function undergoing routine noncardiac surgical procedures, whereas Georgen and colleagues reported the use of balloon pumping specifically in biliary tract surgery.(136,137) The use of intra-aortic balloon pumping provides hemodynamic stability during anesthetic induction and assists in balancing the myocardial oxygen supply:demand ratio preoperatively, perioperatively, and in the critical postoperative period when demands on the heart are particularly high.

Because the first clinical use of intra-aortic balloon pumping was in patients with acute myocardial infarction and cardiogenic shock, it is noteworthy that this historical account of the balloon pump development ends with a recent new indication for counterpulsation also in patients with acute myocardial infarction. Numerous investigations, beginning in the early to mid-1980s, showed the benefits of both thrombolytic therapy and percutaneous transluminal coronary angioplasty as treatments for acute myocardial infarction.(138, 139) Although reperfusion by thrombolytic agents or angioplasty reduces infarct size and eventually improves left ventricular function, the performance of the ischemic myocardium does not immediately improve with reperfusion.(140) Afterload reduction by intra-aortic balloon pumping may be beneficial while awaiting functional recovery. Moreover, because coronary blood flow is often impaired in the early phase of reperfusion, increasing diastolic pressure by counterpulsation may enhance the effects of chemical and mechanical therapies to restore flow.(79, 141) The utility of intra-aortic balloon pumping as an adjunct to reperfusion therapy in acute myocardial infarction has been examined by Ohman et al (87, 142) and also by Ishihara et al (143) This new and exciting indication will be covered, in detail, in a later chapter.

Conclusions

The use of intra-aortic balloon pumping to provide hemodynamic support for seriously ill patients with a wide range of cardiovascular problems has expanded considerably since Kantrowitz, Clauss, Moulopoulos, and their colleagues published their original series. Major technological advances in biomedical materials and balloon design have led to smaller caliber catheters which, in turn, have allowed more patients to be treated with balloon pumps. Other technical advances, especially the widespread use of microprocessors, have resulted in a generation of balloon pump consoles that perform and monitor many of their critical functions automatically and with superb accuracy and dependability. The remaining chapters of this book will greatly expand the information provided in this historical review of the development of the intra-aortic balloon pump.

REFERENCES

1. Kantrowitz A, Kantrowitz A. Experimental augmentation of coronary flow by retardation of the arterial pressure pulse. Surgery 1953;34:678–687.
2. Beck CS. Principles underlying the operative approach to the treatment of myocardial ischemia. Ann Surg 1943;118:788–806.
3. O'Shaughnessy L. Surgical treatment of cardiac ischaemia. Lancet 1937; 232:185–194.
4. Beck CS. The development of a new blood supply to the heart by operation. Ann Surg 1935;102:801–813.

5. Glenn F, Beal JM. The fate of an artery implanted in the myocardium. Surgery 1950;27:841–847.
6. Vineberg AM, Miller WD. An experimental study of the physiological role of an anastomosis between the left coronary circulation and the left internal mammary artery implanted in the ventricular myocardium. Proceedings of the Forum Sessions, 36th Clinical Congress of the American College of Surgeons, Boston, Massachussetts. Philadelphia: WB Saunders; October 1950.
7. Kantrowitz A, McKinnon WMP. The experimental use of the diaphragm as an auxiliary myocardium. Surg Forum 1958;9:266–268.
8. Moreira LFP, Stolf NAG, Bocchi EA, et al. Latissimus dorsi cardiomyoplasty in the treatment of patients with dilated cardiomyopathy. Circulation 1990;82(suppl IV):257–263.
9. Clauss RH, Birtwell WC, Albertal G, et al. Assisted circulation. I. The arterial counterpulsator. J Thorac Cardiovasc Surg 1961;42:447–458.
10. Scheidt S, Collins M, Goldstein J, Fisher J. Mechanical circulatory assistance with the intraaortic balloon pump and other counterpulsation devices. Prog Cardiovasc Dis 1982;25:5576.
11. Lefemine AA, Low HBC, Cohen ML, Harken DE. Assisted circulation. II. The effect of heart rate on synchronized arterial counterpulsation. Am Heart J 1962;64:779–788.
12. Birtwell WC, Soroff HS, Wall M, Bisberg A, Levine HJ, Deterling RA Jr. Assisted circulation: I. An improved method for counterpulsation. Trans Am Soc Artif Intern Organs 1962;8:35–42.
13. Soroff HS, Birtwell WC, Levine HJ, Bellas AE, Deterling RA Jr. Effect of counterpulsation upon the myocardial oxygen consumption and heart work. Surg Forum 1962;13:174–176.
14. Topaz SR. How the balloon pump was conceived: a personal reminiscence. Cardiovasc Dis Bull Texas Heart Inst 1977;4:423–427.
15. Moulopoulos SD, Topaz S, Kolff WJ. Diastolic balloon pumping (with carbon dioxide) in the aorta: A mechanical assistance to the failing circulation. Am Heart J 1962;63:669–675.
16. Kantrowitz A. Introduction of left ventricular assistance. ASAIO Trans 1987;33:39–48.
17. Kantrowitz A, Tjønneland S, Freed PS, Phillips SJ, Butner AN, Sherman JL. Initial clinical experience with intraaortic balloon pumping in cardiogenic shock. JAMA 1968;203:135–140.
18. Kantrowitz A, Tjønneland S, Krakauer JS, Phillips SJ, Freed PS, Butner AN. Mechanical intraaortic cardiac assistance in cardiogenic shock. Arch Surg 1968;97:1000–1004.
19. Griffith GC, Wallace WB, Cochran B, Nerlich WE, Frasher WG. The treatment of shock associated with myocardial infarction. Circulation 1954;9:527–532.
20. Summers DN, Kaplitt M, Norris J, et al. Intra-aortic balloon pumping: hemodynamic and metabolic effects during cardiogenic shock in patients with triple coronary artery obstructive disease. Arch Surg 1969;99:733–738.
21. Bregman D, Kripke DC, Goetz RH. The effect of synchronous unidirectional intra-aortic balloon pumping on hemodynamics and coronary blood flow in cardiogenic shock. Trans Am Soc Artif Organs 1970;16:439–446.

22. Bregman D, Goetz RH. Clinical experience with a new cardiac assist device: the dual-chambered intra-aortic balloon assist. J Thorac Cardiovasc Surg 1971;62:577–591.

23. Buckley MJ, Leinbach RC, Kastor JA, et al. Hemodynamic evaluation of intra-aortic balloon pumping in man. Circulation 1970;41(suppl II):130–136.

24. Dennis C, Moreno JR, Hall DP, et al. Studies on external counterpulsation as a potential measure for acute left heart failure. Trans Am Soc Artif Intern Organs 1963;9:186–191.

25. Soroff HS, Ruiz U, Birtwell WC, Many M, Giron F, Deterling RA. Assisted circulation by external pressure variation. Israel J Med Sci 1969;5:506–514.

26. Jacobey JA, Taylor WJ, Smith GT, Gorlin R, Harken DE. A new therapeutic approach to acute coronary occlusion II. Opening dormant coronary collateral channels by counterpulsation. Am J Cardiol 1963;11:218–227.

27. Watson JT, Platt MR, Rogers DE, Sugg WL, Willerson JT. Similarities in coronary flow between external counterpulsation and intra-aortic balloon pumping. Am J Physiol 1976;230:1616–1621.

28. Johansen KH, DeLaria GA, Bernstein EF. Effect of external counterpulsation in reduction of the myocardial ischemia following coronary artery occlusion. Trans Am Soc Artif Intern Organs 1973;19:419–423.

29. Banas JS, Brilla A, Levine HJ. Evaluation of external counterpulsations for the treatment of angina pectoris. Am J Cardiol 1973;31(abstr):118.

30. Loeb HS, Kahn M, Towne W, Gunnar RM. Effects of external counterpulsation on myocardial ischemia induced by atrial pacing. Circulation 1974;49(suppl II):255–258.

31. Soroff HS, Cloutier CT, Birtwell WC, Begley LA, Messer JV. External counterpulsation: Management of cardiogenic shock after myocardial infarction. JAMA 1974;229:1441–1450.

32. Amsterdam EA, Banas J, Criley JM, et al. Clinical assessment of external pressure circulatory assistance in acute myocardial infarction: Report of a cooperative trial. Am J Cardiol 1980;45:349–356.

33. Lawson WE, Hui JCK, Soroff HS, et al. Efficacy of enhanced external counterpulsation in the treatment of angina pectoris. Am J Cardiol 1992;70:859–862.

34. Lawson WE, Hui JCK, Zheng ZS, et al. Three-year sustained benefit from enhanced external counterpulsation in chronic angina pectoris. Am J Cardiol 1995;75:840–841.

35. DeBakey ME. Left ventricular bypass pump for cardiac assistance. Am J Cardiol 1971;27:3–11.

36. Kantrowitz A, Krakauer J, Rubenfire M, et al. Initial clinical experience with a new permanent mechanical auxiliary ventricle: The dynamic aortic patch. Trans Am Soc Artif Intern Organs 1972;18:159–167.

37. Kantrowitz A, Phillips SJ, Butner AN, Tjønneland S, Haller JD. Technique of femoral artery cannulation for phase-shift balloon pumping. J Thorac Cardiovasc Surg 1968;56:219–220.

38. Wolvek S. The evolution of the intra-aortic balloon: The Datascope contribution. J Biomat Appl 1989;3:527–543.

39. Dunkman WB, Leinbach RC, Buckley MJ, et al. Clinical and hemodynamic results of intraaortic balloon pumping and surgery for cardiogenic shock. Circulation 1972;46:465–477.

40. Scheidt S, Wilner G, Mueller H, et al. Intra-aortic balloon counterpulsation in cardiogenic shock: Results of a co-operative trial. N Engl J Med 1973; 288:979–984.

41. Leinbach RC, Dinsmore RE, Mundth ED, et al. Selective coronary and left ventricular cineangiography during intraaortic balloon pumping for cardiogenic shock. Circulation 1972;45:845–852.

42. Willerson JT, Curry GC, Watson JT, et al. Intraaortic balloon counterpulsation in patients in cardiogenic shock, medically refractory left ventricular failure and/or recurrent ventricular tachycardia. Am J Med 1975; 58:183–191.

43. Baron DW, O'Rourke MF. Long-term results of arterial counterpulsation in acute severe cardiac failure complicating myocardial infarction. Br Heart J 1976;38:285–288.

44. Hagemeijer F, Laird JD, Haalebos MMP, Hugenholtz PG. Effectiveness of intraaortic balloon pumping without cardiac surgery for patients with severe heart failure secondary to a recent myocardial infarction. Am J Cardiol 1977;40:951–956.

45. McEnany MT, Kay HR, Buckley MJ, et al. Clinical experience with intraaortic balloon pump support in 728 patients. Circulation 1978;58(suppl I):124–132.

46. DeWood MA, Notshe RN, Hensley GR, et al. Intraaortic balloon counterpulsation with and without reperfusion for myocardial infarction shock. Circulation 1980;61:1105–1112.

47. Lorente P, Gourgon R, Beaufils P, et al. Multivariate statistical evaluation of intraaortic counterpulsation in pump failure complicating acute myocardial infarction. Am J Cardiol 1980;46:124–134.

48. Pierri MK, Zema M, Kligfield P, et al. Exercise tolerance in late survivors of balloon pumping and surgery for cardiogenic shock. Circulation 1980;62 (suppl I):138–141.

49. Laks H, Rosenkranz E, Buckberg GD. Surgical treatment of cardiogenic shock after myocardial infarction. Circulation 1986;74 (suppl III):11–16.

50. Gold HK, Leinbach RC, Sanders CA, Buckley MJ, Mundth ED, Austen WG. Intraaortic balloon pumping for ventricular septal defect or mitral regurgitation complicating acute myocardial infarction. Circulation 1973;47: 1191–1196.

51. McGee MG, Zillgitt SL, Trono R, et al. Retrospective analyses of the need for mechanical circulatory support (intraaortic balloon pump/abdominal left ventricular assist device or partial artificial heart) after cardiopulmonary bypass: A 44 month study of 14,168 patients. Am J Cardiol 1980;46:135–142.

52. Sturm JT, McGee MG, Fuhrman TM, et al. Treatment of postoperative low output syndrome with intraaortic balloon pumping: Experience in 419 patients. Am J Cardiol 1980;45:1033–1036.

53. Craver JM, Kaplan JA, Jones EL, Kopchak J, Hatcher CR. What role should the intra-aortic balloon have in cardiac surgery? Ann Surg 1979;189:769–776.

54. Beckman CB, Geha AS, Hammond GL, Baue AE. Results and complications of intraaortic balloon counterpulsation. Ann Thorac Surg 1977; 24:550–559.

55. Bregman D, Parodi EN, Edie RN, Bowman FO Jr, Reemtsma K, Malm JR. Intraoperative unidirectional intra-aortic balloon pumping in the management of left ventricular power failure. J Thorac Cardiovasc Surg 1975; 70:1010–1023.

56. Bolooki H, Williams W, Thurer RJ, et al. Clinical and hemodynamic criteria for the use of the intraaortic balloon pump in patients requiring cardiac surgery. J Thorac Cardiovasc Surg 1976;72:756–768.

57. Scanlon PJ, O'Connell J, Johnson SA, Moran JM, Gunnar R, Pifarre R. Balloon counterpulsation following surgery for ischemic heart disease. Circulation 1976;54 (suppl III):90–93.

58. Stewart S, Biddle T, DeWeese J. Support of the myocardium with intra-aortic balloon counterpulsation following cardiopulmonary bypass. J Thorac Cardiovasc Surg 1976;72:109–114.

59. Smith GH, Morgan WE. Experience with counterpulsation in cardiac surgical patients. Br Heart J 1977;39:198–202.

60. Berger RL, Saini VK, Ryan TJ, Sokol DM, Keefe JF. Intra-aortic balloon assist for postcardiotomy cardiogenic shock. J Thorac Cardiovasc Surg 1973;66:906–915.

61. Lamberti JJ, Cohn LH, Lesch M, Collins JJ Jr. Intra-aortic balloon counterpulsation: indications and long-term results in postoperative left ventricular power failure. Arch Surg 1974;109:766–771.

62. Bregman D, Bolooki H, Malm JR. A simple method to facilitate difficult intraaortic balloon insertions. Ann Thorac Surg 1973;15:636–639.

63. Gueldner TC, Lawrence GH. Intraaortic balloon assist through cannulation of the ascending aorta. Ann Thorac Surg 1975;19:88–91

64. Krause AH, Bigelow JC, Page US. Transthoracic intraaortic balloon cannulation to avoid repeat sternotomy for removal. Ann Thorac Surg 1976;21:562–565.

65. Gold HK, Leinbach RC, Sanders CA, Buckley MJ, Mundth ED, Austen WG. Intraaortic balloon pumping for control of recurrent myocardial ischemia. Circulation 1973;47:1197–1203.

66. Levine FH, Gold HK, Leinbach RC, Daggett WM, Austen WG, Buckley MJ. Management of acute myocardial ischemia with intraaortic balloon pumping and coronary bypass surgery. Circulation 1978;58 (supp I):69–72.

67. Weintraub RM, Voukydis PC, Aroesty JM, et al. Treatment of preinfarction angina with intraaortic balloon counterpulsation and surgery. Am J Cardiol 1974;34:809en>814.

68. Weintraub RM, Aroesty JM, Paulin S, et al. Medically refractory unstable angina pectoris. I. Long-term follow-up of patients undergoing intraaortic balloon counterpulsation and operation. Am J Cardiol 1979;43:877–882.

69. Maroko PR, Bernstein EF, Libby P, et al. Effects of intraaortic balloon counterpulsation on the severity of myocardial ischemic injury following acute coronary occlusion. Circulation 1972;45:1150–1159.

70. Kerber RE, Marcus ML, Ehrhardt J, Abboud FM. Effect of intra-aortic balloon counterpulsation on the motion and perfusion of acutely ischemic myocardium. Circulation 1976;53:853–859.

71. Reneman RS, Jageneau AHM, Schaper WKA, Brouwer FAS, VanGervan W. Influence of counterpulsation on collateral circulation after acute occlusion of the left anterior descending coronary artery in dogs. Cardiovasc Res 1972;6:45–53.

72. Saini VK, Hood WB Jr, Hechtman HB, Berger RL. Nutrient myocardial blood flow in experimental myocardial ischemia: Effects of intraaortic balloon counterpulsation and coronary reperfusion. Circulation 1975;52:1086–1090.

73. Sugg WL, Martin LF, Webb WR, Ecker RR. Influence of counterpulsation on aortic right and left coronary blood flow following ligation of the left circumflex coronary artery. J Thorac Cardiovasc Surg 1970;59:345–351.

74. Gill CC, Wechsler AS, Newman GE, Oldham HN Jr. Augmentation and redistribution of myocardial blood flow during acute ischemia by intraaortic balloon pumping. Ann Thorac Surg 1973;16:445–453.

75. Watson JT, Willerson JT, Fixler DE, Sugg WL. Temporal changes in collateral coronary blood flow in ischemic myocardium during intra-aortic balloon pumping. Circulation 1974;50 (suppl II):249–254.

76. Watson JT, Fixler DE, Platt MR, Nall BB, Jett GK, Willerson JT. The influence of combined intra-aortic balloon counterpulsation and hyperosmotic mannitol on regional myocardial blood flow in ischemic myocardium in the dog. Circ Res 1976;38:506–513.

77. Sasayama S, Osakada G, Takahashi M, et al. Effects of intraaortic balloon counterpulsation on regional myocardial function during acute coronary occlusion in the dog. Am J Cardiol 1979;43:59–66.

78. Williams DO, Korr KS, Gewirtz H, Most AS. The effect of intraaortic balloon counterpulsation on regional myocardial blood flow and oxygen consumption in the presence of coronary artery stenosis in patients with unstable angina. Circulation 1982;66:593–597.

79. Fuchs RM, Brin KP, Brinker JA, Guzman PA, Heuser RR, Yin FCP. Augmentation of regional coronary blood flow by intra-aortic balloon counterpulsation in patients with unstable angina. Circulation 1983;68:117–123.

80. Port SC, Patel S, Schmidt DH. Effects of intraaortic balloon counterpulsation on myocardial blood flow in patients with severe coronary artery disease. J Am Coll Cardiol 1984;3:1367–1374.

81. Powell WJ, Daggett WM, Magro AE, et al. Effects of intra-aortic balloon counterpulsation on cardiac performance, oxygen consumption, and coronary blood flow in dogs. Circ Res 1970;26:753–764.

82. Roberts AJ, Alonso DR, Combes JR, et al. Role of delayed intraaortic balloon pumping in treatment of experimental myocardial infarction. Am J Cardiol 1978;41:1202–1208.

83. Laas J, Campbell CD, Takanashi Y, Pick RL, Replogle RL. Failure of intra-aortic balloon pumping to reduce experimental myocardial infarct size in swine. J Thorac Cardiovasc Surg 1980;80:85–93.

84. Leinbach RC, Gold HK, Harper RW, Buckley MJ, Austen WG. Early intraaortic balloon pumping for anterior myocardial infarction without shock. Circulation 1978;58:204–210.

85. O'Rourke MF, Norris RM, Campbell TJ, Chang VP, Sammel NL. Randomized control trial of intraaortic balloon counterpulsation in early myocardial infarction with acute heart failure. Am J Cardiol 1981;47:815–820.

86. Flaherty JT, Becker LC, Weiss JL, et al. Results of a randomized prospective trial of intraaortic balloon counterpulsation and intravenous nitroglycerin in patients with acute myocardial infarction. J Am Coll Cardiol 1985;6:434–446.

87. Ohman EM, Califf RM, George BS, et al. The use of intraaortic balloon pumping as an adjunct to reperfusion therapy in acute myocardial infarction. Am Heart J 1991;121:895–901.

88. Mundth ED, Buckley MJ, DeSanctis RW, Daggett WM, Austen WG. Surgical treatment of ventricular irritability. J Thorac Cardiovasc Surg 1973;66:943–951.

89. Hanson EC, Levine FH, Kay HK, et al. Control of postinfarction ventricular irritability with the intraaortic balloon pump. Circulation 1980;62 (suppl I):130–137.

90. Lefemine AA, Kosowsky B, Madoff I, Black H, Lewis M. Results and complications of intraaortic balloon pumping in surgical and medical patients. Am J Cardiol 1977;40:416–420.

91. McCabe JC, Able RM, Subramanian VA, Gay WA Jr. Complications of intra-aortic balloon insertion and counterpulsation. Circulation 1978;57: 769–773.

92. Alpert J, Bhaktan EK, Gielchinsky I, et al. Vascular complications of intra-aortic balloon pumping. Arch Surg 1976;111:1190–1195.

93. Bregman D, Kripke DC, Cohen MN, Laniado S, Goetz RH. Clinical experience with the unidirectional dual-chambered intra-aortic balloon assist. Circulation 1971;43 (suppl I):82–89.

94. Wolfson S, Karsh DL, Langou RA, Geha AS, Hammond GL, Cohen LS. Modification of intraaortic balloon catheter to permit introduction by cardiac catheterization techniques. Am J Cardiol 1978;41:733–738.

95. Subramanian VA, Goldstein JE, Sos TA, McCabe JC, Hoover EA, Gay WA Jr. Preliminary clinical experience with percutaneous intraaortic balloon pumping. Circulation 1980:62 (suppl I):123–129.

96. Bregman D, Nichols AB, Weiss MB, Powers ER, Martin EC, Casarella WJ. Percutaneous intraaortic balloon insertion. Am J Cardiol 1980;46:261–264.

97. Vignola PA, Swaye PS, Gosselin AJ. Guidelines for effective and safe percutaneous intraaortic balloon pump insertion and removal. Am J Cardiol 1981;48:660–664.

98. Alcan KE, Stertzer SH, Wallsh E, Franzone AJ, Bruno MS, DePasquale NN. Comparison of wire-guided percutaneous insertion and conventional surgical insertion of intra-aortic balloon pumps in 151 patients. Am J Med 1983;75:24–28.

99. Goldberg MJ, Rubenfire M, Kantrowitz A, et al. Intraaortic balloon pump insertion: a randomized study comparing percutaneous and surgical techniques. J Am Coll Cardiol 1987;9:515–523.

100. Alderman JD, Gabliani GI, McCabe CH, et al. Incidence and management of limb ischemia with percutaneous wire-guided intraaortic balloon catheters. J Am Coll Cardiol 1987;9:524–530.

101. Rajai HR, Hartman CW, Innes BJ, et al. Prophylactic use of intra-aortic balloon pump in aortocoronary bypass for patients with left main coronary artery disease. Ann Surg 1978;187:118–121.

102. Vijayanagar R, Bognolo DA, Eckstein PF, Toole JC, Natarajan P, Mukherjee D. The role of intra-aortic balloon pump in the management of patients with main left coronary artery disease. Cathet Cardiovasc Diagn 1981;7:397–401.

103. Kern MJ. Intra-aortic balloon counterpulsation. Cor Art Dis 1991;2: 649–660.

104. Folland ED, Kemper AJ, Khuri SF, Josa M, Parisi AF. Intraaortic balloon counterpulsation as a temporary support measure in decompensated critical aortic stenosis. J Am Coll Cardiol 1985;5:711–716.

105. Alcan KE, Stertzer SH, Wallsh E, DePasquale NP, Bruno MS. The role of intra-aortic balloon counterpulsation in patients undergoing percutaneous transluminal coronary angioplasty. Am Heart J 1983;105:527–530.
106. Hartzler GO, Rutherford BD, McConahay DR, Johnson WL, Giorgi LV. "High-risk" percutaneous transluminal coronary angioplasty. Am J Cardiol 1988;61: 33G–37G.
107. Anwar A, Mooney MR, Stertzer SH, et al. Intra-aortic balloon counterpulsation support for elective coronary angioplasty in the setting of poor left ventricular function: a two center experience. J Inv Cardiol 1990;2:175–180.
108. Voudris V, Marco J, Morice MC, Fajadet J, Royer T. "High-risk" percutaneous transluminal coronary angioplasty with preventive intra-aortic balloon counterpulsation. Cathet Cardiovasc Diagn 1990;19:160–164.
109. Kahn JK, Rutherford BD, McConahay DR, Johnson WL, Giorgi LV, Hartzler GO. Supported "high-risk" coronary angioplasty using intraaortic balloon pump counterpulsation. J Am Coll Cardiol 1990;15:1151–1155.
110. Aguirre FV, Kern MJ, Bach R, et al. Intraaortic balloon pump support during high-risk coronary angioplasty. Cardiology 1994;84:175–186.
111. Reemtsma K, Drusin R, Edie R, Bregman D, Dobelle W, Hardy M. Cardiac transplantation for patients requiring mechanical circulatory support. N Engl J Med 1978;298:670–671.
112. Hardesty RL, Griffin BP, Trento A, Thompson ME, Ferson PF, Bahnson HT. Mortally ill patients and excellent survival following cardiac transplantation. Ann Thorac Surg 1986;41:126–129.
113. Pennington DG, Swartz MT. Mechanical circulatory support prior to cardiac transplantation. Sem Thorac Cardiovasc Surg 1990;2:125–134.
114. Gaul G, Blazek G, Deutsch M, et al. Chronic use of an intraaortic balloon pump in congestive cardiomyopathy. In: Unger F, ed. Assisted Circulation–2. Berlin: Springer-Verlag; 1984; pp 28–37.
115. Mayer JH. Subclavian artery approach for insertion of intra-aortic balloon. J Thorac Cardiovasc Surg 1978;76:61–63.
116. Ruberstein RB, Karhade NV. Supraclavicular subclavian technique of intra-aortic balloon insertion. J Vasc Surg 1984;1:577–578.
117. McBride LR, Miller LW, Naunheim KS, Pennington DG. Axillary artery insertion of an intraaortic balloon pump. Ann Thorac Surg 1989;48:874–875.
118. Kralios AC, Zwart HHJ, Moulopoulos SD, Collan R, Kwan-Gett CS, Kolff WJ. Intrapulmonary artery balloon pumping: assistance of the right ventricle. J Thorac Cardiovasc Surg 1970;60:215–232.
119. Spotnitz HM, Bermen MA, Reis RL, Epstein SE. The effects of synchronized counterpulsation of the pulmonary artery on right ventricular hemodynamics. J Thorac Cardiovasc Surg 1971;61:167.
120. Opravil M, Gorman AJ, Krejcie TC, Mintz L, Michaelis LL, Moran JM. Pulmonary artery balloon counterpulsation for right ventricular failure. Surg Forum 1983;1:282–285.
121. Jett GK, Siwek LG, Picone AL, Applebaum RE, Jones M. Pulmonary artery balloon counterpulsation for right ventricular failure: an experimental evaluation. J Thorac Cardiovasc Surg 1983;86:364–372.
122. Opravil M, Gorman AJ, Krejcie TC, Michaelis LL, Moran JM. Pulmonary artery balloon counterpulsation for right ventricular failure: I. Experimental results. Ann Thorac Surg 1984;38:242–253.

123. Miller DC, Moreno-Cabral RJ, Stinson EB, Shinn JA, Shumway NE. Pulmonary artery balloon counterpulsation for acute right ventricular failure. J Thorac Cardiovasc Surg 1980;80:760–763.

124. Flege JB, Wright CB, Reisinger TJ. Successful balloon counterpulsation for right ventricular failure. Ann Thorac Surg 1984;37:167–168.

125. Moran JM, Opravil M, Gorman AJ, Rastegar H, Meyers SN, Michaelis LL. Pulmonary artery balloon counterpulsation for right ventricular failure: II. Clinical experience. Ann Thorac Surg 1984;38:254–259.

126. Gold JP, Shemin RJ, Disesa VJ, Cohn L, Collins JJ. Balloon pump support of the failing right heart. Clin Cardiol 1985;8:599–602.

127. Gottlieb SO, Chew PH, Chandra N, et al. Portable intraaortic balloon counterpulsation: clinical experience and guidelines for use. Cathet Cardiovasc Diagn 1986;12:18–22.

128. Bellinger RL, Califf RM, Mark DB, et al. Helicopter transport of patients during acute myocardial infarction. Am J Cardiol 1988;61:718–722.

129. Berger RL, Saini VK, Long W, Hechtman H, Hood A Jr. The use of diastolic augmentation with the intra-aortic balloon pump in human septic shock with associated coronary artery disease. Surgery 1973;74:601–606.

130. Mercer D, Doris P, Salerno TA. Intra-aortic balloon counterpulsation in septic shock. Can J Surg 1981;24:643–645.

131. Demas C, Flancbaum L, Scott G, Trooskin SZ. The intra-aortic balloon pump as an adjunctive therapy for severe myocardial contusion. Am J Emerg Med 1987;5:499–502.

132. Lane AS, Woodward AC, Goldman MR. Massive propranolol overdose poorly responsive to pharmacologic therapy: use of the intra-aortic balloon pump. Ann Emerg Med 1987;16:1381–1383.

133. Veasy LG, Blalock RC, Orth JL, Boucek MM. Intra-aortic balloon pumping in infants and children. Circulation 1983;68:1095–1100.

134. Nash IS, Lorell BH, Fishman RF, Baim DS, Donahue C, Diver DJ. A new technique for sheathless percutaneous intraaortic balloon catheter insertion. Cathet Cardiovasc Diagn 1991;23:57–60.

135. Tatar H, Çiçek S, Demirkiliç U, et al. Vascular complications of intraaortic balloon pumping: unsheathed versus sheathed insertion. Ann Thorac Surg 1993;55:1518–1521.

136. Grotz RL, Yeston NS. Intra-aortic balloon counterpulsation in high-risk cardiac patients undergoing non-cardiac surgery. Surgery 1989;106:1–5.

137. Georgen RF, Dietrick JA, Pifarre R, Scanlon PJ, Prinz RA. Placement of intra-aortic balloon pump allows definitive biliary surgery in patients with severe cardiac disease. Surgery 1989;106:808–814.

138. Lavie CJ, Gersh BJ, Chesebro JH. Reperfusion in acute myocardial infarction. Mayo Clin Proc 1990;65:549–564.

139. Topol EJ. Coronary angioplasty for acute myocardial infarction. Ann Intern Med 1988;109:970–980.

140. Braunwald E, Kloner RA. The stunned myocardium: prolonged postischemic ventricular dysfunction. Circulation 1982;66:1146–1149.

141. Grines CL, Topol EJ, Bates ER, Juni JE, Walton JA, O'Neill WW. Infarct vessel status after intravenous tissue plasminogen activator and acute coronary angioplasty: prediction of clinical outcome. Am Heart J 1988;115:1–7.

142. Ohman EM, George BS, White CJ, Kern MJ, Gurbel PA, Freedman RJ, et al. Use of aortic counterpulsation to improve sustained coronary artery patency during acute myocardial infarction: results of a randomized trial. Circulation 1994;90:792–799.

143. Ishihara M, Sato H, Tateishi H, Uchida T, Dote K. Intraaortic balloon pumping as the postangioplasty strategy in acute myocardial infarction. Am Heart J 1991;122:385–389.

2

Physical and Medical Aspects of Inflation Gases: Helium vs Carbon Dioxide*

Raymond R. Shedlick ▪ Gerald A. Maccioli

Inflation gases are employed in intra-aortic balloon pump therapy (IABPT) for two purposes. The "driving gas" powers the pneumatic unit, while the "shuttle gas" moves in and out of the balloon during periods of inflation and deflation. Both helium (He) and carbon dioxide (CO_2) have been used for these actions, although neither gas has proved to be ideal. Each involves tradeoffs in areas of safety or performance. The safety issue revolves around the concern for balloon rupture and subsequent shuttle gas embolism. Carbon dioxide is advantageous in this case due to its superior solubility in blood. The performance issue revolves around shuttle gas response time and the slope of the augmentation curve at rapid heart rates. Helium has the advantage here due to its lower density, which permits improved flow characteristics under the turbulent conditions that exist in an IABP. After a review of these issues, a risk-adjusted recommendation will be made as to which gas is most appropriate for modern IABPT.

The Safety Issue

The primary concern of IABP gas safety is the comparatively uncommon, but potentially lethal, complication of shuttle gas embolization.(1, 2, 10, 12, 17, 19) Furman et al,(5) in a study published in 1971, found that 1 to 3 cc/kg of He, a relatively insoluble gas, was fatal in less than 3 min-

*The authors thank Russell Powell, Clinical Support Specialist, Datascope Corporation, Fairfield, NJ, for his encouragement and support in the preparation of this chapter.

utes. He also demonstrated that as little as 0.5 to 1 cc/kg caused extensive cerebral and coronary artery obstruction and that only 0.25 cc of gas was necessary to occlude a single coronary artery. The proximal location of the balloon to the coronary ostia and the great vessels arising from the , aortic arch makes the selection of a gas with good solubility characteristics a logical choice. Carbon dioxide is more than 70 times more soluble than helium (Table 2.1), 34 times more soluble than air, and dissolves in the blood faster than any known gas. (2, 4, 20)

The significance of solubility becomes apparent when viewing how a bubble of gas behaves once it is introduced into the blood. In general, the gas within a bubble begins to dissolve into the blood, while at the same time gases already present in the blood are moving into the bubble. The gradient initially favors a net transfer out of the bubble until equilibrium is reached. At that point, bubble size remains relatively constant as long as the pressure it is subject to does not change. The more soluble the gas, the faster this process can occur. The initial size of the embolus will also determine how fast it is able to shrink. Large bubbles with their greater surface area-to-volume ratio will not shrink as fast as smaller bubbles, which dissolve easier. In addition, emboli with relatively poor solubility coefficients will remain stable and produce prolonged arterial obstruction. This obstruction begins a cascade of interactions involving platelets and endothelial edema, which can result in distal ischemia.(6) Kunkler and King (7) found that it took five times as much carbon dioxide as air to produce end-organ dysfunction. Their observations illustrate the role of solubility in emboli resolution.

During this experiment the heart and coronary arteries were closely observed. Air and oxygen characteristically produce emboli, which are stable and produce arterial obstruction. Once the air embolus cease to move, it remained permanently in that position. Other air emboli would follow the first and long immobile columns of air would form in the coronary artery. On the other hand, carbon dioxide emboli behave in an entirely different manner. Typically, the bubble of CO_2 gas would rapidly tra-

Table 2.1

Solubility Coefficients	
Gas	*Coefficient*
O_2	0.024
CO_2	0.570
N_2	0.012
He	0.008

Reprinted with permission from Guyton AC. Textbook of Medical Physiology. Eighth ed. Philadelphia: WB Saunders; 1991.

verse the extent of the artery and disappear. As larger amounts were given, the emboli would sometimes pause at a bifurcation and rapidly proceed. When toxic amounts were given, a long column of gas would become immobile, block the artery, and remain essentially as air embolus.

Air is not presently used as an inflation gas in any commercially available IABP. However, it is apparent from the preceding that He—due to its lower solubility—would be even more lethal as an embolus than either air or CO_2. Carbon dioxide's comparative safety advantage as a shuttle gas rests on its significantly higher solubility as long as "nontoxic" amounts of gas did not escape from the balloon.

Gas can be introduced into the circulation from an IABP in several ways:

1. Diffusional losses across the balloon membrane account for approximately 1 cc/h for He and 5 cc/h for CO_2.(8, 18) These losses have not been documented to be detrimental; however, they can nullify some of the theoretical advantages of each gas. Because the diffusion process occurs in both directions, the comparative safety and performance advantages of each gas becomes compromised as the composition of the shuttle gas changes. Periodic purging and refilling are necessary to compensate for this problem in order to maintain the integrity of the shuttle gas.

2. Small balloon leaks are another possible source of emboli. However, there is a scarcity of published information regarding embolization specifically related to leaks of this size. The possible explanations are:
   a. Transmembranous pressures are greater during deflation than inflation. This gradient favors entrainment of blood into the catheter, which is an absolute indication for balloon removal or replacement.
   b. The surface tension at the leak site, that is, the blood/balloon interface, helps impede the loss of shuttle gas.
   c. The total shuttle gas volume is less than the balloon volume so that even at peak inflation the balloon membrane is flaccid.
   d. Leak alarms, loss of augmentation, or the need for frequent refills often herald the loss of balloon integrity, which alerts clinicians to problems with the system before large rents in the balloon occur.

3. Rupture of the balloon is the third and, potentially, the most dangerous method that gas can escape from an IABP. Large tears in the balloon can occur due to manufacturer's defect, improper handling or insertion, and from arteriopathic abrasions. Although the possibility of rupture was noted as early as 1962 by Moulopoulus et al,(16) the incidence of this complication has been shown to be low. Kantrowitz et al,(19) in a study published of 733 insertions, reported a rupture rate of 1.6%.

Stahl et al (1), in a study of 382 insertions, reported a rupture rate of 2.4%. Sutter et al (12) reported a 3.5% rupture rate in 452 insertions, and Alvarez et al (17), a year later, published a retrospective study of 303 insertions, with a rupture rate of 1.7%. These cumulative studies include 1870 patients, and an average rupture rate of 2.2%. A detailed review of the literature reveals that the vast majority of authors feel that this complication is comparatively rare. (2, 3, 4, 8, 10, 11, 13, 14, 15)

From the preceding, several conclusions can be drawn:

1. Gas embolus is an ever-present danger of IABPT, although the incidence is low.
2. Of the three possible ways that shuttle gas can enter the blood, rupture of the balloon is potentially the most dangerous.
3. CO_2 is a safer gas than He based on its superior solubility in blood.
4. The comparative advantage of CO_2 can become marginalized if toxic amounts of gas are released.

The Performance Issue

The ultimate performance of a ventricular assist device such as the IABP must be measured against its ability to reduce the workload of the left ventricle and improve myocardial oxygen supply. In order to function effectively, an IABP should be able to inflate and deflate to its maximum capacity as rapidly as possible at varying heart rates. The ability to do this would optimize its efficiency by increasing coronary blood flow as a result of the rapid rise in aortic end-diastolic pressure during inflation. It would also decrease left ventricular work as a result of its equally rapid deflation, which would cause a fall in presystolic pressure. The steeper rise and fall of the augmentation curve is a function of the shuttle gas response time.

The velocity with which a gas can be introduced into a balloon is dependent on gas volume, pressure, physical characteristics of the balloon catheter, and the vascular resistance against which the balloon must inflate. The configuration of balloon pumps results in turbulent gas flow. Turbulent gas flow offers more resistance than laminar flow. The choice of a shuttle gas, therefore, is dependent on which gas offers the lowest resistance under turbulent conditions. Less resistance means that for a given driving pressure, a greater volume of gas will move into the balloon at a faster rate. Density is the primary determinant of resistance in turbulent flow. A dimensionless calculated figure known as Reynolds' number has been devised to determine when laminar flow converts to turbulent flow. This ratio of viscosity to density is much higher for He than for CO_2, which indicates a later transition to turbulent flow. This has been the basis for the claim that He offers a better response time than CO_2 .

Table 2.2

Viscosity and Density Parameters at 20°C		
Gas	Viscosity (μP)	Density (g/L)
Air	183	1.29
CO_2	149	1.98
He	194	0.18

Reprinted with permission from Hodgman CD, ed. Handbook of Chemistry and Physics. 44th ed. Cleveland, Ohio: The Chemical Rubber Co; 1963, p. 1708.

$$Reynolds\ Number = \frac{vpd}{n}$$

$$where\ v = linear\ velocity\ of\ fluid$$
$$p = density$$
$$d = diameter\ of\ tube$$
$$n = viscosity$$

This assumption has been verified by several authors. Kayser and associates (2), using an AVCO machine, demonstrated that He takes two thirds the time of CO_2 or air to inflate and deflate an intra-aortic balloon (Table 2.3). Tipler and Ghadiali,(21) using a Hoogstraat machine, also found better results with helium (Tables 2.4 and 2.5).

The theoretical significance of helium's superior response time revolves around its ability to quickly inflate and deflate the balloon at rapid heart rates. A relatively slower gas such as CO_2 is not able to distend the balloon as adequately under these conditions. The resulting decrease in the slope of the augmentation curve results in decreased coronary artery blood flow and higher presystolic pressures. Therefore, there is a decrease in the myocardial oxygen supply, while at the same time there is an increase in myocardial oxygen consumption due to the higher afterload and faster rate of left ventricular function. It is for this reason that He is considered to be a better performing shuttle gas than CO_2.

Recommendation

Helium and CO_2 have both been used successfully as shuttle gases. Neither gas has proved to be ideal, because they both involve compromises in the areas of safety and performance. Carbon dioxide's theoretical advantage is due to its superior solubility in blood. However, this advantage can be marginalized if large enough amounts of gas were to escape from the balloon. Helium's advantage lies in its well-documented better response time. These aspects of the gases, however, are not the only variables to consider. This patient population by definition needs a

Table 2.3

Balloon Response Time, Single-Balloon System

Gas	Inflate (ms)	Deflate (ms)
Air	180	180
CO_2	180	180
He	120	120

Reprinted with permission from Kayser KL, Johnson WD, Shore RT. Comparison of driving gases for IABPs. Medical Instrum 1981;15(1;Jan–Feb):51–54.

Table 2.4

Response Time from Maximum Deflation to Maximum Inflation for Gases

Machine	Driving Gas	Time (ms)
Hoogstraat	He	140
Hoogstraat	Air	220
Hoogstraat	CO_2	240

Reprinted with permission from Tipler DR, Ghadiali PE. A comparative study of some technical aspects of three intra aortic balloon pump systems. Intensive Care Med 1981;7:93–98.

Table 2.5

Response Time, from Maximum Inflation to Maximum Deflation for Gases

Machine	Driving Gas	Time (ms)
Hoogstraat	He	60
Hoogstraat	Air	100
Hoogstraat	CO_2	170

Reprinted with permission from Tipler DR, Ghadiali PE. A comparative study of some technical aspects of three intra aortic balloon pump systems. Intensive Care Med 1981;7:93–98.

left ventricular assist device such as the IABP just to maintain a favorable oxygen supply-demand balance. In addition, these patients are subject to more irregular and/or rapid heart rates than the general population. Also, the incidence of balloon rupture with subsequent gas embolization has been shown to be comparatively low. On the basis of these facts, He would appear to be the better choice as a shuttle gas in modern IABPs.

REFERENCES

1. Stahl KD, Tartolani AJ, Nelson RL, Hall MH, Moccio CG, Parnell VA Jr. Intra-aortic balloon rupture. Trans Am Soc Artif Internal Organs 1988; 34:496–499.

2. Kayser KL, Johnson WD, Shore RT. Comparison of driving gases for IABPs. Medical Instrum 1981;15(1:Jan–Feb):51–54.

3. Frederiksen JW, Smith J, Brown P, Zinetti C. Arterial helium embolism from a ruptured intra-aortic balloon. Ann Thorac Surg 1988;46:690–692.

4. Finegan BA, Comm DG. Operative intra-aortic balloon rupture. Can J Anesth 1988;35 (3):297–299.

5. Furman S, Vijayaugar R, Rosenbaum R, McMullen M, Escher DJ. Lethal sequelae of intra-aortic balloon rupture. Surgery 1971;69:121–129.

6. Pierce EC. Specific therapy for arterial air embolism. Ann Thorac Surg 1980;29:300.

7. Kunkler A, King H. Comparison of air, oxygen, and carbon dioxide embolization. Ann Surg 1959;149:97.

8. Author not specified. Intra-aortic balloon pumps. Health Devices 1981;11(1):3–39.

9. Guyton AC: Textbook of Medical Physiology. Eighth ed. Philadelphia: W B Saunders; 1991.

10. McEnany MT, et al. Clinical experience with intra-aortic balloon pump support in 728 patients. Circulation 1978;58(suppl 1):124–132.

11. Rajani R, Keon WJ, Bedard P. Rupture of an intra-aortic balloon: A case report. J Thorac Cardiovasc Surg 1980;79:301–302.

12. Sutter FP, et al. Events associated with rupture of intra-aortic balloon counterpulsation devices. ASAIO Trans 1991;37(1:Jan–Mar):38–40.

13. Weber KT, Janicki J. Intraaortic balloon counterpulsation: A review of physiological properties, clinical results, and device safety. Ann Thorac Surg 1974;17(6):602–631.

14. Author not specified. Intra-aortic balloon pumps. Health Devices 1987; 16:135.

15. Vincente E, Moreno L, Penas L, Diaz L, Fernandez, Loma-Osorio A. Spontaneous rupture of an intra-aortic balloon pump. Intens Care Med 1981;7:311–312.

16. Moulopoulos SD, Topaz S, Kolff WL. Diastolic balloon pumping (with carbon dioxide) in the aorta—a mechanical assistance to the failing circulation. Am Heart J 1962;63:669–675.

17. Alvarez JM, Gares R, Rowe D, Brady P. Complications from intra-aortic balloon counterpulsation: A review of 303 surgical patients. Eur J Cardiothorac Surg 1992;6:530–535.

18. Bolooki H. Clinical application of intra-aortic balloon pump. New York: Futura Publishing; 1984.

19. Kantrowitz A, Tjønneland S, Freed PS, Phillips SJ, Bunter AN, Sherman JL. Clinical experience with intra-aortic balloon pumping in cardiogenic shock. JAMA 1986;203:113–118.

20. Weathersby PK, Homer LD. Solubility of inert gases in biological fluids and tissues: A review. Undersea Biomed Res 1980;7(4):277–296.

21. Tipler DR, Ghadiali. A comparative study of some technical aspects of three intra aortic balloon pump systems. Intensive Care Med 1981;7:93–98.
22. Hodgman CD, ed. Handbook of Chemistry and Physics. 44th ed. Cleveland, Ohio: The Chemical Rubber Co; 1963, p 1708.

3

Physical and Clinical Aspects of Intra-aortic Balloon Pump Catheters

David A. Tate

Intra-aortic Balloon Catheters: Description and Design

Since the first use in humans of intra-aortic balloon pumps in the 1960s,[1] there have been steady improvements in balloon catheter design and function. All available catheters consist of an elongated, "sausage-shaped" balloon of polyurethane or similar material mounted on a vascular platform. The balloon is now almost universally inflated with helium. Carbon dioxide, which had been used in prior years, is now rarely used because of its higher viscosity, which required larger catheter shafts and slower pumping rates. Modern balloon catheters have largely met the challenges of providing effective diastolic augmentation in what Wolvek has described as the "hostile environment" of the atherosclerotic human aorta.[2] As Wolvek has summarized, the balloon material must simultaneously be thin and pliable enough to be tightly wrapped, nondistensible enough to assure appropriate diameter and volume, tough enough to resist abrasion and perforation by spicules of calcium, fatigue-resistant enough to withstand well over 100,000 inflations and deflations per day, and biologically compatible enough that it is not excessively thrombogenic, pyrogenic, or hemolytic.[2] These requirements have essentially been met by all of the intra-aortic balloon catheters that are currently commercially available.

The majority of balloon catheters used in the United States today are manufactured by one of four companies (Arrow-Kontron, Reading,

Penn; Bard Vascular Systems, Haverhill, Mass; Boston-Scientific Cardiac Assist, Natick, Mass; and Datascope, Fairfield, NJ). Products currently available in the United States and their size specifications are shown in Table 3.1. It should be noted, however, that features of specific product lines change frequently and that current specifications should be obtained and verified from company representatives. One of the most important variables regarding balloon selection is size, which will be discussed separately in the following text.

The vast majority of catheters used today are double lumen, with one lumen allowing for gas transport and the other central lumen allowing atraumatic placement over a J-tip guidewire as well as central aortic pressure monitoring after the balloon is placed. Thus, double-lumen catheters allow for safer placement of the balloon and also make it unnecessary to establish a separate arterial line to obtain a waveform for balloon pump timing. In the event of difficult passage, the dual-lumen catheter also allows the possibility of careful injection of a small amount of radiographic contrast agent to rule out the possibility of having entered a false lumen.(3) Other design features that vary somewhat by product line are many and include composition of the catheter shaft, flexibility of the catheter shaft, balloon material, balloon cycle time, folded versus wrapped membrane, and the presence of distal and proximal radiopaque markings. In addition, catheters from one company are often compatible with drive consoles from another, but this should always be verified by company representatives.

Intra-aortic Balloon Catheters: Size Selection

Balloon sizing has been empirically derived but follows from two general principles. The first is that the balloon should ideally lie from just below the left subclavian artery to just above the renal arteries. The second is that the diameter should provide maximal displacement of volume without distending the aorta itself.

Placement of the balloon "too high," above the left subclavian artery, has the obvious potential disadvantage of compromising cerebral blood flow, either directly or via atheromatous or thrombotic embolism. Placement "too low," below the renal arteries, has the effect of compromising renal blood flow and, therefore, renal function. In addition, the abdominal aorta tapers significantly below the origins of the celiac and renal arteries and also tends to have much more calcific atheroma than the thoracic aorta. The size mismatch between the balloon and aorta at this level therefore greatly increases the risk of aortic disruption. The calcific plaque, moreover, greatly increases the risk of balloon rupture. The vast majority of balloon leaks occur in the lower few inches of the balloon, presumably reflecting the decreased aortic diameter and increased calci-

Table 3.1

Intra-aortic Balloon Catheter Size Specifications

Balloon Catheter Type	Balloon Volume (cc)	Balloon Diameter (mm)	Balloon Length (mm)	Catheter Size (Fr)	Folded/Wrapped Membrane Size
Arrow-Kontron					
Stainless-Steel Central Lumen	30	15	228	8	10.5
	40	16	260	9	10.5
	50	18	260	10	10.5
Flexi-Cath	40	16	262	9.5	10.5
Sheathless	40	16	262	9	10.5
ArrowFlex	40	16	262	9.5	10.5
NarrowFlex	40	16	262	8.0	9.5
Bard Vascular Systems					
Rediguard	30	15.6	242	9	10.7
	40	16.25	275	9	10.7
Redifurl	30	15.6	242	9	10.7
	40	16.25	275	9	10.7
	50	18.3	275	11	12.5
TaperSeal	30	15.6	242	9	10.7
	40	16.25	275	9	10.7
	50	18.3	275	11	12.5
Boston-Scientific (Cardiac Assist)					
930	30	15	210	9	10
940	40	15	275	9	10
Sensation 30	30	15	204	9	10
Sensation 40	40	17	220	9.5	10
Datascope					
Percor STAT-DL (optional	34	14.7	219	9.5	9.5
sheathless)	40	15	263	9.5	9.5
	50	16.3	269	10.5	10.5

fication in the abdominal aorta. For all of these reasons, it has long been recognized that ideal balloon placement is from just below (1–2 cm) the left subclavian to just above the renal arteries. Because the distance from the subclavian origin to the celiac and renal origin will vary according to patient size (primarily height), most manufacturers now make adult balloons in three sizes.

For any given length of balloon, the volume of the balloon will then follow as a function of the balloon's inflated diameter. Specifically, the volume will be proportional to the square of the inflated diameter. Ideally, one wants to displace as much blood volume as possible for optimal hemodynamic effect, but if the balloon diameter exceeds that of the aorta, there is no additional physiologic gain, and there is an increased risk of aortic trauma and balloon disruption. In 1971, Weikel and colleagues(4) studied 169 adult aortograms and found mid-thoracic aortic diameters ranging from 16 to 30 mm, with 90% of patients having aortic diameters greater than 19 mm.(4) No male patients had diameters less than 18 mm, and although there was a trend toward greater aortic diameter with increased age and weight, there was too much scatter for these criteria to be predictive. Thus, the sizes of commercially available balloon pump catheters are now generally between 14 and 16.5 mm. This translates to volumes between 30 and 50 cc, with most adults using balloons with 40 cc. These sizes allow effective counterpulsation but minimize the risks of trauma to the aortic wall, disruption of the balloon, and hemolysis.

As a practical matter, decisions regarding size selection will generally be guided by the devices and recommendations available from the specific manufacturers. This is appropriate in that the companies' product lines have been developed in order to conform with the observations as discussed previously.

Datascope offers three balloon sizes for the adult. The 34-cc balloon (219-mm length, 14.7- mm diameter) is recommended for patients who are less than 5'4" in height. The 40-cc balloon (263-mm length, 15.0-mm diameter) is recommended for patients between 5'4" and 6 ft in height. The 50-cc balloon (269-mm length, 16.3-mm diameter) is recommended for patients more than 6 ft in height. In practice, we have noted that the larger 50-cc balloons are relatively infrequently used and generally reserved for patients well over 6 feet in height. This probably reflects conservative medical judgment and is reasonable, although it should be noted that there is an approximately 15% difference in augmentation between the 50-cc and 40-cc balloons.

Arrow-Kontron balloon catheters are available in 30-cc (228-mm length, 15-mm diameter); 40-cc (260- and 262-mm length, 16-mm diameter); and 50-cc (260-mm length, 18-mm diameter). Bard balloon catheters are available in 30-cc (242-mm length, 15.6-mm diameter); 40-cc (275-mm length, 16.25-mm diameter); and 50-cc (275-mm length, 18.3-mm diameter). Boston-Scientific Cardiac Assist balloon catheters are available in a 30-cc size (204- and 210-mm length, 15-mm diameter) and a 40-cc size (220- and 275-mm length, 15- and 17-mm diameter).

A second and somewhat independent sizing issue is the size of both the catheter shaft and the vascular sheath through which the balloon catheter may be inserted. Adult catheter shaft sizes presently available range from 8 to 11 French (see Table 3.1). However, the outer diameter of the sheath through which the balloons are passed is usually at least 2 French sizes larger than the catheter shaft itself. Also, in some designs the wrapped or folded membrane size is up to 2 French larger than the shaft itself, thus requiring a larger sheath. The shaft and membrane sizes for available products are also shown in Table 3.1.

Because limb ischemia remains a major limitation of intra-aortic balloon pumping (5, 8, 9) and is caused in large part simply by a size mismatch of the catheter-sheath system in diseased femoral and iliac arteries, techniques for sheathless insertion have recently been developed.(6, 7) With this technique, indwelling catheter area can be reduced by approximately 30%. Initial studies suggest that this translates to a decreased incidence of limb ischemia, with little if any increase in bleeding complications. In an initial report by Nash and colleagues, using a Datascope product, sheathless insertion was associated with only a 10% incidence of limb ischemia sufficient to warrant discontinuation of counterpulsation or surgical intervention.(6) This compared favorably to a 27% incidence in historical controls at the same institution,(8) and there was no associated increase in bleeding complications. The authors pointed out that by using a sheathless technique, indwelling catheter diameter was reduced from 3.8 mm to 3.2 mm, and cross-sectional area was reduced from 11.5 mm^2 to 7.9 mm^2, a 31% reduction. In a subsequent retrospective analysis by Tatar et al,(7) using a Kontron product, sheathless insertion was associated with a vascular complication rate of only 8.8% as compared with 25.9% with conventional insertion techniques. Thus, the initial experience with sheathless balloon catheter insertion has been favorable, and it is becoming widely accepted. This technique is likely to have a particularly beneficial role in patients at highest risk for limb ischemia such as small and/or female patients and those with peripheral vascular disease or diabetes.(9) Although there does appear to be a learning curve,(6) the technique of sheathless insertion is relatively simple. With generous spreading of subcutaneous tissues and adequate predilatation of the catheter track, sheathless insertion can be accomplished in the vast majority of patients.

Two manufacturers (Arrow-Kontron and Datascope) presently provide balloon catheters specifically designed for sheathless insertion. These catheters have a tapered or "ballistic" tip, which may be advanced into the femoral artery directly over a guidewire following adequate predilatation. The Datascope product has no stepdown in size between the folded balloon and catheter shaft. The Arrow-Kontron catheter does have a stepdown and is therefore equipped with a short premounted hemostasis device with a bottleneck taper from 9.5 to 11 French that can be used in the event of problems with hemostasis. The Arrow-Kontron product has a siliconized stainless-steel central lumen, and the Datascope product has a tack-weld at the proximal end of the balloon to enhance pushability.

REFERENCES

1. Kantrowitz A, Tjønneland S, Freed PS, Phillips SJ, Butner AN, Sherman JL. Initial clinical experience with intraaortic balloon pumping in cardiogenic shock. JAMA 1968;203:135–140.
2. Wolvek S. The evolution of the intra-aortic balloon: The Datascope contribution. J Biomater Appl 1989;3:527–542.
3. Kantrowitz A, Cardona RR, Freed PS. Percutaneous intra-aortic balloon counterpulsation. Crit Care Clin 1992;8(4):819–837.
4. Weikel AM, Jones RT, Dinsmore R, Petschek HE. Size limits and pumping effectiveness of intra-aortic balloons. Ann Thorac Surg 1971;12(1):45–53.
5. Skillman JJ, Kim D, Baim DS. Vascular complications of percutaneous femoral cardiac interventions. Arch Surg 1988;123:1207–1212.
6. Nash IS, Lorell BH, Fishman RF, Baim DS, Donahue C, Diver DJ. A new technique for sheathless percutaneous intraaortic balloon catheter insertion. Cathet Cardiovasc Diagn 1991;23:57–60.
7. Tatar H, Cicek S, Demirkilic U, et al. Vascular complications of intraaortic balloon pumping: unsheathed versus sheathed insertion. Ann Thorac Surg 1993;55:1518–1521.
8. Alderman JD, Gabliani GI, McCabe CH, et al. Incidence and management of limb ischemia with percutaneous wire-guided intraaortic balloon catheters. J Am Coll Cardiol 1987;9:524–530.
9. Gottlieb SO, Brinker JA, Borkon M, et al. Identification of patients at high risk for complications of intraaortic balloon counterpulsation: A multivariate risk factor analysis. Am J Cardiol 1984;53:1135–1139.

4

Triggering and Timing of the Intra-aortic Balloon Pump

Warner J. Lucas ▪ Mark P. Anstadt

Introduction

The process toward understanding the complex interaction between intra-aortic balloon dynamics and cardiovascular dynamics has taken place over the past 25 years. Early studies elucidated the effects on balloon-assisted circulation as a result of variations in device stroke volume, pumping rate, and position of the device in the aorta. Nerz et al (1), in 1979, found that continuation of inflation into early systole produced maximum benefits to coronary blood flow, and that more effective assist was provided with larger balloon volumes. However, since 1970 it has been appreciated that the single most important determinant of effective balloon-assisted circulation is the synchronization of IABP inflation-deflation to the cardiac cycle,(2) that is, the timing of the intra-aortic balloon pump (IABP).

The properly timed IABP will achieve three goals: improve myocardial oxygen delivery by increasing coronary perfusion pressure, reduce cardiac work by decreasing systolic blood pressure (afterload), and thereby improve forward blood flow in those patients with impaired cardiac function. Although early recommendations for balloon timing attempted to achieve these goals using fairly empiric criteria, subsequent work has provided a scientific basis for current recommendations. Furthermore, technologic advancements have provided closed-loop control systems for using these objective criteria to automatically optimize IABP timing.(3–7)

Control Systems: The Quest

The ultimate goal of an automated IABP system requires the availability of easily measurable parameters, which represent dependable indicators of cardiac performance and myocardial viability. These parameters are integrated into a feedback mechanism that allows subtle adjustments in inflation and deflation to optimize the myocardial oxygen supply-demand relationship. Compounding this challenge are the inevitable alterations in myocardial function and electrophysiology that exist during cardiac failure.(8, 9)

Functional characteristics of the cardiovascular system are constantly changing, particularly in the failing heart. Because the IABP itself imparts some change in measured parameters, it was recognized that automatic control is desirable to maximize performance. The earliest attempts at automatic control were open-loop systems that employed empirically controlled algorithms. To be reliable, an automatic system must include some mechanism for evaluating the control algorithm's effectiveness. Early systems (10–12) measured hemodynamic parameters or combinations thereof for the generation of a performance index. A system analysis was employed that adjusted device parameters while measuring the resulting hemodynamics and their calculated effect on the performance index.

In 1971, Kane et al (10) used mean systolic pressure (MSP), mean diastolic pressure (MDP), and end-diastolic pressure (EDP) as part of a derived performance index. The index was then used to measure the effects of changing delays between aortic valve closure and balloon inflation as well as the duration of balloon inflation. Although underscoring the value of proper timing, this approach had limited application when faced with changing states of ventricular function. Others based performance indices on cardiac output, coronary flow, tension time index,(11) and endocardial viability ratio.(12) Although useful, a common criticism of all such systems was the subjective nature of the derived indices.

The principal goal of balloon counterpulsation is to improve the balance between myocardial oxygen consumption and supply. One feasible approach is to assume that MDP is a good index of coronary blood flow (CBF), and hence oxygen availability. He et al (13) measured CBF in dogs instrumented with IABP and demonstrated a strong correlation between MDP and CBF. Additional theoretical models as well as animal studies have underscored the strong relationship between MDP and coronary blood flow.(14) These studies serve to validate Barnea's performance index which, based on differences between MDP and peak systolic pressure (PSP),(15) assumed that all regulatory mechanisms of the failing heart are exhausted, and that coronary blood flow has a linear relationship with coronary perfusion pressure (MDP). However, improvements in MDP and CBF alone do not necessarily imply improvements in myocardial oxygen supply-demand ratios.

To satisfy the principal requisite of a favorable myocardial oxygen balance, Smith et al in 1991 used a performance index incorporating PSP and MDP.(5) Previous work demonstrated a good correlation between MDP and coronary perfusion (and hence O_2 delivery) over a specified range of IABP drive parameters. In addition, PSP exhibited a high correlation with cardiac O_2 consumption. Therefore, Smith et al proposed a performance index based on PSP and MDP, and confirmed earlier work (14) that maximum coronary perfusion occurred when balloon inflation coincided with end-systole. Timing of deflation, however, involved a critical balance between inflation, which dictates the degree of coronary perfusion augmentation (ie, increases in myocardial oxygen delivery) and deflation, which predicates the effectiveness of afterload reduction (ie, decreases in myocardial oxygen consumption). Using MDP and PSP as indicators of oxygen delivery and oxygen consumption, respectively, it was postulated that a performance index could be reliably based on their difference. A control system for the IABP was subsequently developed that measured PSP and MDP from an aortic pressure tracing, digitized the signal, and calculated the performance index. The system subsequently varied deflation time to maximize the index. Initially, the operator selected inflation time and entered the modifying constants for the measured parameters. The system's internal controller then automatically performed consecutive step-limited adjustments in deflation time, with subsequent aortic pressure waveform analysis. The operator also had the ability to weight entered variables to alter the influence of the IABP on either increasing oxygen delivery or decreasing oxygen demand.

There is general agreement and sound physiological basis for the ideal point of balloon inflation: at end-systole, immediately after the aortic valve closes. Determining the optimal point of deflation, however, is more challenging and the subject of some controversy. Because maximizing coronary perfusion and optimizing left ventricle unloading require *different* deflation points, there is no consensus on optimal timing of balloon deflation. To say simply that balloon deflation should occur before the next systole or before the volume displacement phase of systole appears insufficient. For example, Barnea et al (14) in 1990 demonstrated that improved performance was obtained when balloon deflation began before end-diastole and continued into early systole. Furthermore, Kantrowitz et al (7) reported on a series of patients who were treated with a closed-loop automatic IABP that provided the usual end-systole inflation point and a deflation period that bridged end-diastole and early systole. Clinical results demonstrated a favorable outcome using such a timing scheme.

Although it is clear that balloon inflation can be properly timed to optimize myocardial oxygen delivery, the timing of balloon deflation that best decreases left ventricular oxygen consumption is less well-defined. It is unequivocal that deflation before ventricular ejection creates a low pressure effect in the proximal aorta, which reduces afterload and peak systolic pressure. The resultant net decrease in oxygen consumption is difficult to quantitate. However, PSP is directly related to ventricular wall stress, and the relationship between wall stress and oxygen consumption is well established.

Although O_2 consumption may be reduced with afterload reduction, improper timing (late deflation) can greatly increase oxygen consumption. To avoid this problem, present recommendations to decrease ventricular workload include adjusting IABP deflation to achieve maximal reduction in end-diastolic aortic pressure (EDP). This approach is supported by classic studies done in isolated heart models, which demonstrate good correlation between oxygen consumption and EDP.(16)

In addition to the timing of IABP inflation and deflation, some consideration must be given to the efficiency of the inflation-deflation process. Jaron et al (17), in 1983, demonstrated a lumped-parameter model which, among other things, illustrated that optimization of IABP support required *instantaneous* inflation to maximum volume at end systole and subsequent instantaneous, complete deflation at end-diastole. Although such ideal mechanics are not feasible in clinical practice, expedient balloon actuation has clearly proved most beneficial.

Clinical Considerations

Triggering

Triggering of balloon counterpulsation requires the existence of a predictable, reproducible, and reliable event. The trigger event is the signal that IABP systems use to predict all other relevant components of the cardiac cycle; the trigger marks a timepoint to which balloon inflation and deflation are indexed. Most commonly, the R wave of the electrocardiogram (ECG) serves as the triggering event. Although the more sophisticated systems offer additional triggering capabilities such as the arterial pressure waveforms, ventricular or atrioventricular pacer spikes. The IABP can also trigger independent of the patient at a physiologic rate that the operator selects.

ECG Trigger

Electrocardiogram triggering requires detection of a QRS complex with a specific minimum displayed voltage (eg, 120 µV). The ECG signal is fed to a microprocessor that discriminates the R wave and integrates the signal with operator set timing adjustments. The system thus relays control signals to the device's pneumatic system, which actuates the balloon in accordance with these parameters. Because the presence of external electrical interference (eg, pacemaker spikes and electrosurgical interference) can seriously interfere with reliable trigger event detection, many devices (eg, Datascope System 97 Intra-Aortic Balloon Pump, Datascope Corporation, Fairfield, NJ) have incorporated filters for maintaining proper triggering and timing capabilities under such adverse conditions. If pacer spikes are present, many devices have algorithms for recognition and morphologic discrimination based on signal amplitude and duration. Thereby, rejection of pacer spikes becomes automatic while functioning in the ECG trigger mode.

Pacer Trigger

In instances where patients are paced with ventricular or atrioventricular sequential pacers, a pacer trigger mode may be employed. In such cases, the ventricular pacer spike functions as the trigger event. However, for the IABP to be maximally effective while operating in this mode, patients should be continually paced to prevent missed assisted beats during periods of non-paced intrinsic electrical activity.

Because intraoperative use of balloon counterpulsation is common, IABPs must be equipped with electrosurgical noise suppression capabilities that prevent unwanted triggering from chaotic electrical signals. In addition, while triggering in the pacer mode, balloon pumping will be suspended during operation of the electrosurgical unit. Because pacemaker function may likewise be inhibited during use of electrosurgical devices, the balloon operator must be particularly observant while operating in the pacer trigger mode. In such cases, if possible, it is best to use ECG or arterial pressure waveform as the trigger event.

Pressure Trigger

A positive deflection of the arterial waveform can serve as the trigger event in the pressure trigger mode. Usually, a minimum deflection of 15 mm Hg is required, but some IABP systems have adjustable pressure thresholds. The trigger signal may be obtained from the arterial pressure measured through the central lumen of the balloon or from other arterial cannulation sites. When the pressure trigger mode is used, care must be taken to ensure that balloon deflation occurs *before* the upstroke of the successive systole. Because such systems rely on a prominent upstroke, an unwanted diminution of systolic pressure caused by late deflation may result in a missed trigger event. In addition, because irregular rhythms generate a variety of arterial waveform morphologies, triggering in the pressure mode should be reserved for instances when ECG signals are inadequate and cardiac rhythm is fairly uniform.

Internal Trigger

In those instances when the patient fails to generate either a reliable ECG signal or an arterial pressure waveform, most IABP devices provide an asynchronous balloon pumping mode triggered from an internally generated signal. The trigger rate is adjustable over a physiologic range. For instance, during cardiopulmonary resuscitation, the balloon may be used in an attempt to augment coronary perfusion pressure. To prevent adverse effects, the device will monitor for intrinsic ECG activity and will deflate the balloon on R wave detection. As soon as reliable electrocardiographic activity is detected, the device should be returned to the ECG trigger mode.

Timing

Proper intra-aortic balloon timing interfaces balloon actuation with the mechanical events of the cardiac cycle. The resultant counterpulsation will augment aortic pressures during diastole and reduce peak pressures during systole (Fig. 4.1). Optimal augmentation of pressure during diastole is dependent not only upon timing of the inflation but also on balloon position, speed of balloon inflation, volume of blood displacement, the compliance of the central arterial system, and aortic valve competence.

Timing of balloon deflation presupposes a desire to decrease myocardial oxygen demand during systole. Deflation of the balloon just before the ventricular ejection phase creates a sudden diminution of aortic volume that reduces pressure within the aortic root. This balloon-induced reduction in aortic pressure effectively decreases left ventricular afterload, and

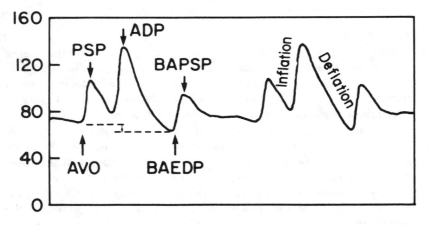

Figure 4.1. *Arterial tracing of properly timed 2:1 balloon assist. Note inflation at dicrotic notch, with resultant significantly augmented diastolic pressure. Also note the lowered balloon-assisted end-diastolic pressure (BAEDP) and lowered balloon-assisted peak systolic pressure (BAPSP), which represents decreased afterload following balloon deflation. Reprinted with permission from Maccioli GA, Lucas WJ, EA Norfleet. The Intra-Aortic Balloon Pump: A Review. J Cardiothoracic Anesthesia 1988;2(3):365–373.*

consequently diminishes myocardial workload (Fig. 4.2). It has long been known that afterload (pressure work) is significantly more costly in terms of myocardial oxygen consumption than cardiac output (volume work).(18) Many feel that afterload reduction is the most beneficial effect of the IABP on the failing heart.(19,20)

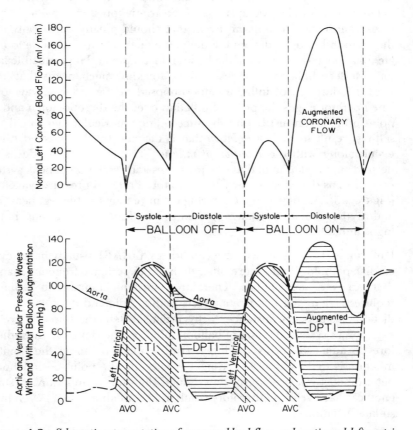

Figure 4.2. *Schematic representation of coronary blood flow and aortic and left ventricular pressure waves, with and without intra-aortic balloon augmentation. (Top panel) Left coronary blood flow changes during the cardiac cycle. Peak flows occur during diastole, when intraventricular pressures are decreased. Balloon augmentation of diastolic aortic root pressure produces further increases in coronary blood flow. (Bottom panel) TTI (tension time index) and DPTI (diastolic pressure time index) illustrated as the area under the left ventricular and aortic pressure curves during systole and diastole, respectively. Proper balloon inflation during diastole augments diastolic pressure and consequently increases coronary perfusion pressure as well as improves the relationship between myocardial oxygen supply and demand (DPTI:TTI ratio). Reprinted with permission from Maccioli GA, Lucas WJ, Norfleet EA. The Intra-Aortic Balloon Pump: A Review. J Cardiothoracic Anesthesia 1988;2(3):365–373.*

Proper operation in IABP is a prerequisite to its beneficial effects. Safe and effective application of these operator-dependent principles requires a fundamental understanding of the cardiac cycle combined with a few technical skills. First, the operator must be able to determine the beginning of diastole. The mechanical event on the arterial pressure tracing indicating end-systole is the dicrotic notch, which represents closure of the aortic valve. Second, the operator must be able to determine the beginning of systole. The upstroke of the arterial pressure waveform indicates ventricular ejection, an event that should ideally occur only after the balloon has been deflated. Finally, the operator must be able to initiate inflation and deflation of the balloon in a rapid and reproducible fashion. Modern balloon consoles provide tracking mechanisms that highlight the duration of inflation superimposed on the arterial waveform. The operator aligns the point of inflation over the dicrotic notch and the point of deflation just before the succeeding ventricular ejection. These settings result in *balloon inflation* that is dictated by the selected trigger event, along with the *duration of inflation*. Proper timing produces the desired augmentation of diastolic pressures and reduction of peak systolic pressures, as demonstrated by the monitored arterial pressure waveform (Figure 4.3). As long as the triggering event remains stable (eg, heart rate and rhythm remain unchanged), the need for further adjustments in timing is unlikely.

Unfortunately, patients who are candidates for IABP usually have severe cardiac pathology, and more often than not experience frequent changes in heart rate and rhythm. Therefore, constant attention to timing is required. Changing heart rate affects both systole and diastole in a predictable fashion. For instance, tachycardia shortens diastole to a greater extent than systole. Timing of balloon inflation and deflation must therefore be adjusted correspondingly. During manual timing the point of inflation is tied by time to a trigger event, and the point of deflation is determined by a previously determined duration of inflation. A shortened cardiac cycle will therefore result in late inflation and an even more so late deflation.

Manual Timing

Timing adjustments on IABP consoles may be performed in either of two modes: *manual* or *automatic*. Manual controls allow adjustments in the interval between the recognized trigger event and balloon inflation. In this mode, the operator examines the point of inflation superimposed over the arterial waveform while fine-tuning the delay interval to synchronize inflation with diastole. The control for deflation essentially determines the duration of inflation. Changes in position of the deflation point are made by varying the inflation interval. In fact, after the initial timing is manually set, future adjustments in the point of inflation will

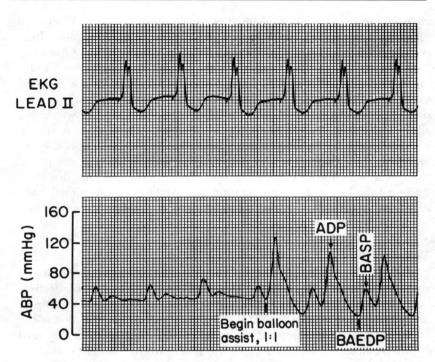

Figure 4.3. *Electrocardiogram and arterial pressure tracing in a patient with left ventricular failure following coronary artery bypass grafting. Initiation of IABP assist resulted in increased systemic blood pressure and successful weaning from cardiopulmonary bypass. Note significant diastolic augmentation and lowered afterload, reflected by decreased peak systolic pressure. Abbreviations: ADP = augmented diastolic pressure; BAEDP = balloon-assisted end-diastolic pressure; BASP = balloon-assisted systolic pressure; ABP = arterial blood pressure. Reprinted with permission from Maccioli GA, Lucas WJ, Norfleet EA. The Intra-Aortic Balloon Pump: A Review. J Cardiothoracic Anesthesia 1988;2(3):365–373.*

correspondingly shift the deflation point in the same direction as the inflation point adjustment. Consequently, any single timing adjustment should include re-evaluation of all timing parameters.

Automatic Timing

To aid in proper timing and simplify clinical application, manufacturers have developed an operating mode that automatically adjusts timing under conditions of varying rate and rhythm. The internal algorithms that allow such automatic adjustments are largely proprietary, but presumably use R-R intervals to estimate alterations in heart rate as well as systolic and diastolic durations. For instance, when heart rates increase, manually preset inflation points relative to the R wave are automatically adjusted, and the duration of inflation (deflation point) is readjusted to reflect a predicted shortened diastolic phase. In clinical situations where cardiac rhythm is irregular, detection of a "premature" R wave results in a default deflation of the balloon. Without automatic adjustments in timing, the operator must remain particularly vigilant in an effort to respond to rate and rhythm variations. Failure to adjust timing parameters in such situations could result in ineffective diastolic augmentation or worse yet, allow prolonged balloon inflation, with its attendant deleterious effects. The automatic timing mode adjusts the inflation and deflation of the balloon as it tracks changes in heart rate and rhythm, which compensates for changes in duration of systole and diastole. One should note, however, that even devices with automatic timing capabilities require initial manual determination of inflation and deflation points before automatic timing can be effectively used.

The Future

The future of balloon-assisted circulation lies in the further development and clinical application of automated closed-loop systems that effectively use monitored patient hemodynamic parameters to facilitate support of the failing heart. If the past 25 years of progress is any indication of the future, the next quarter century should witness great strides toward improved circulatory assist devices and more effective patient care.

REFERENCES

1. Nerz AR, Myerowitz PD, Blackshear PL Jr. A simulation of the dynamics of counterpulsation. J Biomech Eng Trans ASME 1979;101(2):105–111.
2. Jaron D, Tomecek J, Freed PS, Welkowitz W, Fich S, Kantrowitz A. Measurement of ventricular load phase angle as an operating criterion for in series assist devices: Hemodynamic studies using intra-aortic balloon pumping. Trans Am Soc Artif Intern Organs 1970;16:466–471.
3. Jaron D, Moore TW, He P. Control of intraaortic balloon pumping: Theory and guidelines for clinical applications. Ann Biomed Eng 1985;13(2):155–175.
4. Zelano JA, Li JK, Welkowitz W. A closed-loop control scheme for intraaortic balloon pumping. IEEE Trans Biomed Eng 1990;37(2):182–192.
5. Smith B, Barnea O, Moore TW, Jaron D. Optimal control system for the intra-aortic balloon pump. Med Biol Eng Comput 1991;29(2):180–184.
6. Barnea O, Smith BT, Dubin S, Moore TW, Jaron D. Optimal controller for intraaortic ballon pumping. IEEE Trans Biomed Eng 1992;39(6):629–634.
7. Kantrowitz A, Freed PS, Cardona RR, et al. Initial clinical trial of a closed loop, fully automatic intra-aortic balloon pump. ASAIO J 1992;38(3):M617–M621.
8. Jaron D, Ohley W, Kuklinski W. Efficacy of counterpulsation: Model and experiment. Trans Am Soc Artif Intern Organs 1979;25:372–377.
9. Kuklinski WS, Ohley WJ, Jaron D. Computer simulation of optimized intraaortic balloon pumping. Proc 33rd ACEMB 1980;22:165.
10. Kane GR, Clark JW, Bourland HM, Hartley CJ. Automatic control of intra-aortic balloon pumping. Trans Am Soc Artif Intern Organs 1971;17:148–152.

11. Williams MJ, Rubin JW, Ellison RG. Experimental determination of optimum performance of counterpulsation assist pumping under computer control. Comput Biomed Res 1977;10(6):545–559.
12. Jablkowski, Serafin J. Parameter optimization of intra-aortic balloon pumping. Trans ISAO/IFAC Symp 1980;2:245–266.
13. He P, Dubin SE, Moore TW, Jaron D. Guidelines for optimal control of intraaortic balloon pumping. ASAIO J 1984;7(4):172–179.
14. Barnea O, Moore TW, Dubin SE, Jaron D. Cardiac energy considerations during intraaortic balloon pumping. IEEE Trans Biomed Eng 1990; 37(2):170–181.
15. Barnea O, Smith B, Moore TW, Jaron D. An optimal control algorithm for intra-aortic balloon pumping. 11th International Conference. IEEE Engineering in Medicine and Biology Society: Seattle, Washington; 1989.
16. Monroe G, French GN. Left ventricular pressure-volume relationships and myocardial oxygen consumption in the isolated heart. Circ Res 1961;9: 362–374.
17. Jaron D, Moore TW, He P. Theoretical considerations regarding optimization of cardiac assistance by intraaortic balloon pumping. IEEE Trans Biomed Eng 1983;30(3):177–185.
18. Sarnoff SJ, Braunwald E, Welch GH Jr, Case RB, Stainsby WN, Macrus R. Hemodynamic determinants of oxygen consumption of the heart with special reference to the Tension-Time Index. Am J Physiol 1958;192:148–156.
19. Buckley MJ, Leinbach RC, Kaston JA, et al. Hemodynamic evaluation in intraaortic balloon pumping in man. Circ 1970;45(suppl 2):130.
20. Rose EA, Marrin CAS, Bregman D, et al. Left ventricular mechanics of counterpulsation and left heart bypass, individually and in combination. J Thorac Cardiovasc Surg 1979;77:127.

5

Intra-aortic Balloon Pump Utilization

PART A

IABP Therapy in Patients Undergoing Noncardiac Surgery

Robin E. Boineau • Brian Annex

Introduction

Myocardial ischemia and perioperative myocardial infarctions are the most frequent causes of major perioperative morbidity and mortality in patients undergoing noncardiac surgery.(1–4) The cardiotoxicity previously associated with general anesthetic agents has markedly improved with the use of newer pharmacologic agents and improvements in other anesthetic techniques. However, myocardial ischemia can still occur during and after surgery from several inciting factors, including: hypotension, tachycardia (due to pain and neuroendocrine responses), extubation, anemia, shifts of fluids between extravascular and intravascular compartments, and an enhancement in the coagulation system. Although the risk of postoperative myocardial ischemia appears lower when patients can undergo coronary revascularization before surgery,(5) situations arise when this is not feasible, possible, or desirable. These clinical situations include: coronary artery disease that is not amenable to surgery or coronary angioplasty; multivessel coronary artery disease when emergent noncardiac surgery is needed; or severe comorbid diseases, which make the patient a poor candidate for coronary artery bypass surgery. In these situations, the elective placement of an intra-aortic balloon pump (IABP) is an additional therapeutic option that may be able to decrease the risk or consequences of peri- and postoperative myocardial ischemia in selected patients.

Myocardial Ischemia as Risk for Postoperative Complications

Myocardial ischemia is the major risk for postoperative mortality in patients undergoing noncardiac surgery. In a landmark study, Goldman et al (2,6) retrospectively evaluated 1001 consecutive patients who were more than 40 years of age and underwent noncardiac surgical procedures to identify the major risk factors associated with postoperative cardiac death. These risk factors identified included: a recent myocardial infarction, congestive heart failure, arrhythmias, aortic stenosis, age, urgency of surgery, and intraoperative hypotension lasting longer than 10 minutes. Perhaps more important was the fact that the authors were able to assign a relative point score to each of these variables to estimate the risk of a postoperative cardiac event (Table 5A.1). Patients were then assigned to a "Class" based on their point score (Table 5A.2), and the risk of a life-threatening cardiac event or death was calculated for each class. Cardiac risks were greatest in Classes III and IV patients. The risk of a life-threatening cardiac complication was 11% (Class III) and 22% (Class IV), and the risk of death was 22% (Class III) and 56% (Class IV). In contrast, the risk for a life-threatening complication was 5% (Class II) and 0.7% (Class I), and the risk of death was 2% (Class II) and 0.2% (Class I).

To extend and evaluate Goldman's criteria, Zeldin (7) performed a prospective analysis in 1140 patients undergoing general anesthesia for noncardiac surgery. All patients were evaluated postoperatively to determine the incidence of life-threatening cardiac complications (cardiogenic pulmonary edema, myocardial infarction, and witnessed ventricular tachycardia) and cardiac death (arrhythmias and low cardiac output). The incidence of life-threatening cardiac complications and death was: 0.5 and 0.2% for the Class I patients (n = 590); 2 and 1% for the Class II patients (n = 453); 11 and 4% for the Class III patients (n = 74); and 4 and 26% for the Class IV patients (n = 23), respectively for each class. Qualitatively, these findings were quite similar to Goldman's study.

The Goldman and Zeldin studies applied to all patients undergoing noncardiac surgery, and therefore these patients may be considered a low-risk group. In contrast, Detsky et al (8,9) studied 455 patients referred for a cardiology evaluation before noncardiac surgery, which suggested that the referring physician suspected the patient to be at risk for a cardiac event. The authors prospectively developed a modified risk index to determine the probability of a perioperative cardiac event. The Detsky criteria and class point assignments are shown in Table 5A.3. Compared with the Goldman study, the Detsky criteria added information on symptoms of coronary artery disease. The likelihood ratios of a perioperative cardiac event was 0.42 for Class I patients, 3.58 for Class II patients, and 14.93 for Class III patients. A likelihood ratio less than 1 indicates a

Table 5A.1

Goldman's Criteria for Risk of Cardiac Complications in Patients Undergoing Noncardiac Surgery

Points	Finding
11	S_3 gallop or elevated JVP (>12 cm H_2O)
10	Myocardial infarction within 6 months
7	Rhythm other than sinus or PACs
7	PVCs > 5 mon documented
5	>70 y
4	Emergency surgery
3	intraperitoneal, intrathoracic, or aortic surgery
3	Significant aortic stenosis
3	Po_2 < 60 mm; Pco_2 > 50; K+ < 3.0 mEq/L; HCO3 < 20 mEq/L; BUN > 50 mg/dL; Cr > 3.0 mg/dL; chronic liver disease., elevated transaminases, or patient bedridden secondary to noncardiac etiology

Key: *JVP = jugular venous pressure; PACs = premature atrial contractions; PVCs = premature ventricular contractions; Po_2 = partial pressure of oxygen; PCO_2 = partial pressure of carbon dioxide; K+ = potassium; Hco_3 = bicarbonate; BUN = blood urea nitrogen; Cr = creatinine.*

Adapted from Goldman L, Caldera DL, Southwick FS, et al. Cardiac risk factors and complications in non-cardiac surgery. Medicine 1978;57:357–370; and Goldman L, Caldera DL, Nussbaum SR, et al. Multifactorial index of cardiac risk in noncardiac surgical procedures. N Engl J Med 1977;297:845–850.

Table 5A.2

Goldman's Class for Risk of Cardiac Complications in Patients Undergoing Noncardiac Surgery

Class	Points
I	0–5
II	6–12
III	13–25
IV	26+

Adapted from Goldman L, Caldera DL, Southwick FS, et al. Cardiac risk factors and complications in non-cardiac surgery. Medicine 1978;57:357–370; and Goldman L, Caldera DL, Nussbaum SR, et al. Multifactorial index of cardiac risk in noncardiac surgical procedures. N Engl J Med 1977;297:845–850.

below-average risk, and a ratio greater than one indicates a greater-than-average risk for that patient undergoing surgery. It is important to note that these criteria assume that if a surgical procedure can be postponed and the patient stabilized, then the operative risk will be reduced.

Table 5A.3

	Detsky Criteria and Class Assignments
Points	Criteria
20	Critical AS suspected
20	Canadian Cardiovascular Society Class 4 angina
10	Canadian Cardiovascular Society Class 3 angina
10	Unstable angina < 6 mo
10	Myocardial infarction ≤ 6 mo
5	Myocardial infarction > 6 mo
10	Alveolar pulmonary edema, within 1 week
	Alveolar pulmonary edema, ever
10	Emergency surgical procedure
5	Rhythm other than sinus
5	> 5 PVCs/min documented
5	Poor general medical status (as defined per Goldman index)
Detsky Class I	0–15 points
Detsky Class II	16–30 points
Detsky Class III	> 30 points

Key: *AS = aortic stenosis; PVC = premature ventricular contractions.*

Coronary Revascularization and the Risk of Perioperative Ischemia

Using the Coronary Artery Surgery Study (CASS) registry, Foster et al (5) retrospectively evaluated 1600 patients who had undergone noncardiac surgery and coronary angiography (excluding individuals with cardiomyopathies, valvular and congenital heart disease) between July 1, 1974 and May 31, 1979. These individuals were divided into three groups: Group I (n = 399) had no angiographic evidence of coronary artery disease (CAD); Group II (n = 743) had angiographic evidence of significant CAD and underwent coronary artery bypass graft (CABG) before noncardiac surgery; Group III (n = 458) had CAD documented, but had noncardiac surgery without coronary revascularization. For the entire population the operative mortality was 1.3% but the highest mortality, 2.4%, occurred in the patients in Group III. This excess mortality in the patients who did not undergo coronary revascularization before their noncardiac surgery was statistically significant compared with the 0.5 and 0.9% mortality rates in Groups I and II patients. It is important to note that this study involved individuals who survived coronary artery bypass surgery and the individuals not surviving bypass surgery were not included in the analysis. Also this study was retrospective and it was not possible to determine how the decision to perform bypass surgery might have influenced the overall outcomes. Nevertheless, this study appears to support the idea that when ischemic heart disease is treated before noncardiac surgery there is less myocardial ischemia and its associated complications in these patients.

Percutaneous transluminal coronary angioplasty (PTCA) is another revascularization strategy to consider in patients with coronary artery disease who need noncardiac surgery. Indeed, PTCA may be viewed as a potentially useful revascularization strategy for these patients because compared with coronary artery bypass surgery, PTCA has a shorter recovery time and has virtually no effect on other organ systems, such as the pulmonary or renal systems. PTCA is considered the treatment of choice for patients with single vessel coronary artery disease and preserved left ventricular function.(10) In many situations results from multi-vessel PTCA have been comparable to those obtained from CABG.(11) PTCA is also often effective for patients not considered candidates for bypass surgery.(12) Only one study has evaluated PTCA as a revascularization strategy before noncardiac surgery. Huber et al (13) studied 50 patients who underwent PTCA before their noncardiac surgery and found that the frequency of a perioperative infarction was 5.6% and mortality was 1.9%. Unfortunately, the study was not randomized and did not have a control group for comparison. The study also excluded five patients from the analysis who did not have successful angioplasty because the cardiologists were either unable to cross the lesion (n=3) or there were complications related to the PTCA and the patients underwent CABG before noncardiac surgery. There are no studies available to determine the best time to perform surgery after PTCA. However, because most angioplasty complications, such as acute myocardial infarctions and abrupt closures, occur within the first 3 days (> 80% within first 24 hours) surgery should be deferred at least 4 days whenever feasible.(14)

Mechanisms of IABP Protection

Although coronary artery revascularization before elective or urgent noncardiac surgery may confer protection against postoperative myocardial infarctions, there are circumstances in which revascularization is not possible. A series of conventional medical therapies can be used to decrease the risk, severity, or sequelae of postoperative myocardial ischemia. These include aspirin, β-blockers, nitrates, and in some cases, calcium channel blockers. Also, by using data obtained from invasive monitoring (pulmonary artery catheters and arterial lines) changes in preload and afterload, blood pressure, acid-base status, and oxygenation, which can precipitate myocardial ischemia, can be quickly identified and treated. In sedated patients, changes in the pulmonary capillary wedge pressure or blood pressure may be the first sign of myocardial ischemia.

The use of an IABP is another therapeutic option in high-risk patients. The IABP has several features that operate to assist the heart.(15–18) The IABP expands during systole and thereby decreases afterload by decreasing volume in the aorta and improving the aortic compliance. This in turn, lowers end-systolic pressure, left ventricular end-systolic volume, and end-diastolic aortic pressure, which results in decreased myocardial demand. The decrease in afterload can improve left ventricular stroke volume and the ejection fraction. The decrease in myocardial demand can reduce the incidence of ischemia. The IABP also augments myocardial blood flow by increasing diastolic aortic pressures and lowering the corresponding left ventricular diastolic pressure. The decreased wall tension and reduction in afterload translate to a reduction in myocardial oxygen demand. Finally, cerebral circulation may be increased with the IABP, and although renal perfusion may not increase, the urine output does increase.

The ability of the IABP to prevent ischemia or to ameliorate the consequences of ischemia in patients with coronary artery disease is well established.(19–20) In patients undergoing PTCA, the IABP has been shown to improve vessel patency rates in the setting of an angioplasty dissection.(21) The IABP also appears useful in high-risk patients with an acute myocardial infarction.(22) In the setting of a total coronary occlusion, the IABP can improve collateral blood flow.(23) The precise mechanisms by which IABP therapy can confer protection for patients in these settings or as an adjunctive therapy for patients undergoing noncardiac surgery is unknown.

IABP Therapy for Noncardiac Surgery: Literature Review

There are no randomized studies evaluating the IABP in individuals undergoing noncardiac surgery. A number of case reports have evaluated the use of an IABP to prevent postoperative complications in a high-risk population. The studies all involved individuals with known coronary disease that did not undergo coronary revascularization because they were considered inoperable; had a severe co-existent disease process (ie, malignancy); or a noncardiac procedure that needed to be done on an emergent basis. Due to the myriad of clinical situations in which the use of the IABP is described, each of the reports will be reviewed.

Grotz et al (24) reported on three patients (ages 57, 67, and 75 years) with multivessel coronary artery disease and mildly impaired left ventricular function who required emergent noncardiac surgery. Two of three patients presented with acute myocardial infarction and the third had accelerating angina. All three patients had an IABP placed for perioperative support. The first patient required a subtotal gastrectomy and Biliroth I anastomosis for gastrointestinal (GI) bleeding. The IABP was removed on postoperative Day 3. The second patient underwent an exploratory laparotomy and repair of an incarcerated parastomal hernia for a small bowel obstruction that did not respond to conservative decompression. His IABP was removed on postoperative Day 2. The third patient underwent surgery to remove a frontal lobe meningioma after the patient presented with evolving neurologic changes and a CT scan showing left frontal mass with increasing perihemispheric edema. None of the patients had evidence of perioperative cardiac complication.

Georgen et al (25) reported on 15 patients ages 49 to 75 years, who presented with chronic (n = 6) or acute cholecystitis (n = 9). All were Goldman Class IV with a mean ejection fraction of 21% (± 3%) and all but one were men. Two patients had experienced a myocardial infarction within the prior 2 months. All patients underwent a cholecystectomy. In addition to the cholecystectomy, 4 patients also underwent an intraoperative cholangiogram; 1 patient had a common bile duct exploration; and one patient had a cystgastrostomy for a pancreatic pseudocyst. Two of the patients died of arrhythmias in the postoperative period (Days 1 and 9). The remainder were alive at follow-up (3 months–7 years). Of these 13 patients, 3 went on to have orthotopic heart transplantation. The authors noted a significant decrease in the pulmonary capillary wedge pressure (24 ± 3 to 16 ± 2 mm Hg) and pulmonary artery pressures with IABP placement. The IABPs were removed Days 1 to 9, with the mean at Day 3. One patient had leg pain that required removal of the IABP. The Goldman criteria predicted a mortality rate of 50%, but, in this small population, the observed mortality rate was only 13%.

Siu and co-workers (26) evaluated eight men with a mean age of 70 (range, 47–82) who were considered high-risk for surgery with one or more of the following criteria: (1) Goldman Classes III or IV; (2) New York Heart Association Classes 3 or 4 (unstable) angina; (3) left main or multivessel coronary artery disease with evidence of ischemia on radionucleotide imaging, or 4) angiographically documented multivessel coronary artery disease with history of hemodynamic instability during previous noncardiac surgery. All patients were placed on intravenous nitroglycerin and invasive monitoring and an IABP was used. Four patients had heparin or low molecular weight dextran while the IABP was in place. Six patients had the IABP removed by postoperative Day 2, and one patient had IABP removed emergently because of vascular compromise. The other two patients had the IABP removed Days 4 and 11 postoperatively. There were three "early" postoperative cardiac events (1 myocardial infarction, 1 episode of severe pulmonary edema/CHF, and 1 fatal gastrointestinal bleed following emergent femoral thrombectomy with heparin therapy). There were three late noncardiac deaths.

One patient developed sepsis and multisystem organ failure and died 4 weeks after surgery. One patient died of respiratory failure 4 weeks after requiring emergent coronary artery bypass surgery with mitral valve replacement, on the 5th postoperative day following the noncardiac surgery. The third patient died 6 weeks postoperatively from pneumonia and respiratory failure.

Bonchek and Olinger (27) investigated the outcome of three patients with severe coronary artery disease undergoing a thoracotomy for a malignancy work-up. All patients were considered poor candidates for bypass surgery because of the unclear nature of the thoracic lesions. All patients had an IABP placed and there were no significant cardiac problems or complications from the IABP. Two patients were discharged on Days 5 and 10 postoperatively, but one patient was not able to have a curative resection, developed multiple noncardiac problems and died 3 weeks later.

An approach to severe combined symptomatic carotid artery and coronary artery disease was reported by Myers et al.(28) Five patients were scheduled for a carotid endarterectomy (CEA) with an IABP placed pre-CEA, followed by a neurologic evaluation post-CEA and by coronary artery grafting 24 hours later. This approach resulted from reluctance of cardiothoracic surgeons to perform coronary artery bypass grafting in these patients with severe symptomatic carotid artery stenosis. Neither pressors nor vasodilators were used intraoperatively. All the CEA procedures were uneventful. The IABPs were removed 3 to 4 days after coronary artery surgery. There were no cardiac complications, but one patient required a femoral embolectomy and repair of a false femoral aneurysm. At 14 month follow-up, none of the patients were experiencing angina or neurologic symptoms.

Foster et al (29) reported on three patients requiring urgent abdominal surgery that used IABP therapy. The first patient, age 57, had undergone removal of left ventricular aneurysm and had biventricular failure with a low cardiac output. The IABP was used to improve his cardiac output during removal of a hypernephroma. He had only mild liver failure postoperatively. The second patient was an 88-year-old man with severe aortic stenosis (AS) and two syncopal episodes who needed an urgent colectomy. He had extensive diverticulosis, which required transfusion of 32 units over 21 days. He had an IABP placed and was sent to surgery during a recurrent bleeding episode. The third patient was a 64-year-old man with left ventricular failure and severe mitral regurgitation. He underwent mitral valve replacement (MVR) and had low cardiac output postoperatively. He then developed melena and evidence of blood in his nasogastric tube aspirates. He required 15 units of blood over 72 hours and was taken to surgery for vagotomy and pyloroplasty for a bleeding duodenal ulcer. There was no evidence of a perioperative myocardial infarction in any of these patients. The third patient died 1 month after MVR from renal failure.

Miller and Hall (30) discussed a patient who required an emergency gastrectomy following an upper GI bleed 13 days after an anterior wall myocardial infarction. He had required 20 transfusions over 4 days. The IABP use was interrupted during use of the cautery secondary to noise interference with triggering of the electrocardiogram (ECG). During this period, the patient developed an increased wedge pressure (16–26 mm Hg) and hypotension (systolic blood pressure to 95). The patient had an IABP removed after 18 hours because of poor circulation to his leg but was eventually sent home, on the 16th postoperative day.

Georgeson et al (31) discussed three patients (ages 63–70) with significant coronary artery disease and required surgery for treatment of acute cholecystitis, debulking of ovarian tumor with exploratory laparotomy, and an esophagogastrectomy for treatment of esophageal cancer. The first patient had an ischemic cardiomyopathy and prosthetic aortic valve. The second and third patients were considered to have inoperable coronary artery disease. The first patient developed ventricular ectopy and ischemic mitral regurgitation intraoperatively and was treated with lidocaine and nitroglycerin. The second patient tolerated an episode of a postoperative supraventricular tachycardia with no elevation in cardiac enzymes. The third patient developed an atrial tachycardia with ischemia on ECG postoperatively. This was associated with a small elevation in total cardiac enzymes but no major hemodynamic instability. Notably, all the patients were discharged home without any further problems.

There are obvious limitations in applying this nonrandomized data to understand the actual efficacy of the IABP. Overall, the patients in the previously mentioned studies appeared to have a lower mortality rate than would otherwise be expected from their complex medical risk profile. Moreover, in situations where ischemia was present, the ischemia may have been better tolerated hemodynamically. Whether this is due to the effectiveness of the IABP or random chance is uncertain.

IABP Therapy for Patients Undergoing Noncardiac Surgery

Georgeson et al (31) used a method, termed decision analysis, to evaluate the efficacy of IABP therapy in patients undergoing noncardiac surgery. The first step in this process involved evaluating the efficacy of the IABP in preventing postoperative myocardial infarction. To do this, the authors cited a large study of patients who underwent coronary artery bypass surgery in which 75 patients had IABP and 55 patients did not have an IABP placed before surgery (although all patients were good candidates for IABP therapy). A perioperative myocardial infarction occurred in 5 (6.7%) of 75 patients with IABP compared with 16 (29%) of 55 patients without an IABP. The efficacy of the IABP in preventing myocardial infarctions was determined to be 0.77. [Efficacy = 1–(frequency of event with treatment ÷ frequency of the event without treatment), where frequency of event with treatment was 0.067 (6.7%), and frequency of the event without treatment was 0.29 (29%).]

The next step in the analysis attempted to account for the fact that an IABP placement is not always successful and can have associated complications. The probability a patient would have an unsuccessful insertion of IABP was determined to be 6%, and the probability of death from insertion of IABP was 0.672 from complications such as infection, bleeding, or surgical repair.

The next step of the decision analysis was to assign a utility value to each outcome. The utility value is a subjective number given to an outcome based on just how favorable or unfavorable the event may be. A utility value of one indicates a perfect outcome. Zero is the value assigned to death. Amputation was assigned a value of 0.58, a vascular complication was assigned a value of 0.95, and a myocardial infarction, 0.90. The lower the value, the greater the estimated loss of function. The utility values were used in calculating outcome effects on quality of life. The life expectancy was adjusted based on demographic parameters (mortality statistics for age, gender, and race), and then modified using the utility values to determine a quality-adjusted life expectancy for an individual patient. The life expectancy was the reciprocal of the sums of the values contributing to an increased mortality rate.

The authors then applied this data to different clinical scenarios that were evaluated using different predictive models. Of note, different degrees of benefit were predicted depending on which model was used. However, overall the gain in quality-adjusted life expectancy (or quality-adjusted life years) was limited in patients with "severe" cardiac or comorbid disease processes, because of a short life expectancy associated with that process. If the patients had a longer life expectancy, they would derive greater benefit from use of IABP intraoperatively.

Due to the uncertainty of the value assigned for efficacy and the importance of this value as the first step in the decision analysis, Georgeson et al (31) plotted patients in various classes against various efficacies of the IABP. He used the probability of a life-threatening cardiac event for a given class and the corresponding probability of death (given a life-threatening event). From this data, Georgeson extrapolated that individuals in Detsky Classes II and III (and undergoing "major" noncardiac surgery) and Goldman Class IV would benefit from use of the IABP, even if the efficacy is less than 10%. In summary, he concluded that individuals with less than 2% risk of death with noncardiac surgery would not benefit from use of the IABP because of higher associated complication risks. If the individual's probability of life-threatening complications for a noncardiac surgical procedure is greater than 29%, then prophylactic placement of the IABP is beneficial.

Summary

In summary, cardiac morbidity and mortality is the leading cause of death following noncardiac surgery. Previous nonrandomized studies have indicated that patients' outcome is improved when coronary revascularization is performed before noncardiac surgery, particularly if a major procedure in high-risk individuals is planned. The greatest risk factors associated with cardiac mortality include advanced age, congestive heart failure, emergent procedure, and recent myocardial infarction. Patients with multiple risk factors for coronary artery disease, especially those with a history of changing angina, should be evaluated before surgery for risk stratification. This evaluation should include exercise testing and possibly coronary angiography. Patients with accelerating or unstable angina should be considered for possible PTCA or CABG before noncardiac surgery. When PTCA or CABG is not a feasible alternative, then the use of a prophylactic IABP should be considered in the high-risk cardiac patient. This method appears to reduce the risk of cardiac morbidity and mortality in the appropriately selected patient population. However, randomized studies should be performed to access the benefits of the IABP in the setting of noncardiac surgery.

REFERENCES

1. Mangano DT, Browner WS, Hollenberg M, et al. Association of perioperative myocardial ischemia with cardiac morbidity and mortality in men undergoing noncardiac surgery. N Engl J Med 1990;323:1781–1788.
2. Goldman L, Caldera DL, Southwick FS, et al. Cardiac risk factors and complications in non-cardiac surgery. Medicine 1978;57:357–370.
3. Rao TLK, Jacobs KH, El-Etr AA. Reinfarction following anesthesia in patients with myocardial infarction. Anesthesiology 1983;59:499–505.
4. Mangano DT. Perioperative cardiac morbidity. Anesthesiology 1990; 72:153–184.
5. Foster ED, Davis KB, Carpenter JA, et al. Risk of noncardiac operation in patients with defined coronary disease: The Coronary Artery Surgery Study (CASS) Registry Experience. Ann Thorac Surg 1986;41:42–49.
6. Goldman L, Caldera DL, Nussbaum SR, et al. Multifactorial index of cardiac risk in noncardiac surgical procedures. N Engl J Med 1977;297:845–850.
7. Zeldin RA. Assessing cardiac risk in patients who undergo noncardiac surgical procedures. Can J Surg 1984;27:402–404.
8. Detsky AS, Abrams HB, McLaughlin JR, et al. Predicting cardiac complications in patients undergoing non-cardiac surgery. J Gen Intern Med 1986; 1:211–219.

9. Detsky AS, Abrams HB, Forbath N, et al. Cardiac assessment for patients undergoing noncardiac surgery. Arch Intern Med 1986;146:2131–2134.
10. Parisi AF, Folland ED, Hartigan P, et al. A comparison of angioplasty with medical therapy in the treatment of single-vessel coronary artery disease. N Engl J Med 1992;326:10–16.
11. Hamm CW, Reimers J, Ischinger T, et al. A randomized study of coronary angioplasty compared with bypass surgery in patients with symptomatic multivessel coronary disease. N Engl J Med 1994;331:1037–1043.
12. Morrison DA, Barbierre C, Cohan A, et al. Percutaneous transluminal coronary angioplasty for rest angina pectoris requiring intravenous nitroglycerin and intraaortic balloon counterpulsation. Am J Cardiol 1990;66:168–171.
13. Huber KC, Evans MA, Bresnahan JF, et al. Outcome of noncardiac operations in patients with severe coronary artery disease successfully treated preoperatively with coronary angioplasty. Mayo Clin Proc 1992;67:15–21.
14. Detre KM, Holmes Dr Jr, Holubkov R, et al. Incidence and consequences of periprocedural occlusion: the 1985–1986 NHLBI Percutaneous Transluminal Coronary Angioplasty Registry. Circulation 1990;82:739–750.
15. Nanas JN, Moulopoulos SD. Counterpulsation: historical background, technical improvements, hemodynamic and metabolic effects. Cardiology 1994;84:156–167.
16. Underwood MJ, Firmin RK, Graham TR. Current concepts in the use of intra-aortic balloon counterpulsation. Br J Hospl Med 1993;50:391–397.
17. Weber KT, Janicki JS. Intraaortic balloon counterpulsation. Ann Thorac Surg 1974;17:602–636.
18. Urschel CW, Eber L, Forrester J, et al. Alteration of mechanical performance of the ventricle by intraaortic balloon counterpulsation. Am J Cardiol 1970;25:546–551.
19. Port SC, Shantilal P, Schmidt DH. Effects of IABP counterpulsation on myocardial blood flow in patients with severe coronary artery disease. J Am Coll Cardiol 1984;3:1367–1374.
20. D'Agostino RS, Baldwin JC. Intra-aortic balloon counterpulsation: present status. Compr Ther 1986;12:47–54.
21. Ohman EM, George BS, White CJ, et al. Use of aortic counterpulsation to improve sustained coronary artery patency during acute myocardial infarction. Circulation 1994;90:792–799.
22. Ohman EM, Califf RM, George BS, et al. The use of intraaortic balloon pumping as an adjunct to reperfusion therapy in acute myocardial infarction. Am Heart J 1991;121:895–901.
23. Kern MJ, Aguirre F, Bach R, et al. Augmentation of coronary blood flow by intra-aortic balloon pumping in patients after coronary angioplasty. Circulation 1993;87:500–511.
24. Grotz RL, Yeston NS. Intra-aortic balloon counterpulsation in high-risk cardiac patients undergoing noncardiac surgery. Surgery 1989;106:1–5.
25. Georgen RF, Dietrick JA, Pifarre R, et al. Placement of intra-aortic balloon pump allows definitive biliary surgery in patients with severe cardiac disease. Surgery 1989;106:808–814.
26. Siu SC, Kowalchuk GJ, Welty FK, et al. Intra-aortic balloon counterpulsation support in the high-risk cardiac patient undergoing urgent noncardiac surgery. Chest 1991;99:1342–1345.

27. Boncheck LI, Olinger GN. Intra-aortic balloon counterpulsation for cardiac support during noncardiac operations. J Thorac Cardiovasc Surgery 1979;78:147–149.

28. Myers SI, Valentine RJ, Esterera A, et al. The intra-aortic balloon pump, a novel addition to staged repair of combined symptomatic cerebrovascular and coronary artery disease. Ann Vasc Surg 1993;7:239–242.

29. Foster ED, Olsson CA, Rutenburg AM, et al. Mechanical circulatory assistance with intra-aortic balloon counterpulsation for major abdominal surgery. Ann Surg 1976;183:73–76.

30. Miller MG, Hall SV. Intra-aortic balloon counterpulsation in high-risk cardiac patient undergoing emergency gastrectomy. Anesthesiology 1975;42: 103–105.

31. Georgeson S, Coombs AT, Eckman MH. Prophylactic use of the intra-aortic balloon pump in high-risk cardiac patients undergoing noncardiac surgery: A decision analytic view. Am J Med 1992;92:665–678.

5

PART B

Use of Intra-aortic Balloon Pump Therapy in the Cardiac Catheterization Laboratory

Robert J. Applegate ▪ Gregory A. Braden ▪ Michael A. Kutcher

Introduction

The use of intra-aortic balloon pump (IABP) therapy in patients with ischemic heart disease has increased tremendously in the past 20 years. This expanded use has paralleled the growth and development of Interventional Cardiology. During these years the cardiac catheterization laboratory has evolved from a pure diagnostic service to a multidimensional role that includes the percutaneous revascularization of patients with ischemic heart disease. In its earliest use intra-aortic balloon pump therapy was often a last ditch effort to stabilize a patient with peri-infarction angina, or to support a patient with cardiogenic shock complicating an acute myocardial infarction. Anecdotal reports chronicled isolated successes, however, there were no data or experience to support more widespread use of this modality. Moreover, insertion of the balloon pump was initially performed via a surgical cutdown with the inherent complications of vascular repair. The development of a percutaneous insertion technique is one factor that led to the greater use of intra-aortic balloon pump therapy since the early 1980s. Other factors that led to a more widespread use of intra-aortic balloon pump therapy included the successful development of coronary angioplasty technology, and a growing experience in management of patients with acute ischemic syndromes and hemodynamic instability, which allowed application of interventional techniques to a high-risk group of patients. Although angioplasty could be more broadly applied, use in patients with severe left ventricular (LV) dysfunction, or coronary arteries subserving a critical amount of remaining viable myocardium, became limiting factors. At the same time techno-logical improvements in the percutaneous femoral delivery of angioplas-ty equipment paralleled the adaptation of the intra-aortic balloon pump to permit safe percutaneous placement in the cardiac catheterization lab-oratory. The adjunctive use of support measures including intra-aortic balloon pump therapy in the cardiac catheterization laboratory provided a stable hemodynamic platform in patients with severe LV dysfunction or critical myocardium at jeopardy to allow safer and more effective con-sideration of percutaneous revascularization options in high-risk patients unsuitable for surgical revascularization. In this chapter we hope to examine use of intra-aortic balloon pump therapy in a wide variety of patients with ischemic and non-ischemic heart disease under both elec-tive and emergency conditions in the cardiac catheterization laboratory (Table 5B.1).

Use in Ischemic Heart Disease

Use of Intra-aortic Balloon Pump during Elective Percutaneous Revascularization

High-Risk Angioplasty

In the late 1980s, as experience with angioplasty grew, patients with severe LV dysfunction, or with a stenosis subtending a critical portion of remaining viable myocardium, became limiting factors to the widespread application of percutaneous transluminal coronary angioplasty (PTCA). Hartzler and colleagues,(28) and others (4,29) identified patients under-going elective angioplasty who were at high risk for significant peri-pro-cedural morbidity and mortality. In 6500 patients undergoing elective coronary angioplasty between 1980 and 1987, peri-procedural complica-tions were assessed.(28) As can be seen in Table 5B.2, reduced LV func-tion, severe three-vessel or left main coronary artery disease were associ-ated with a several fold increase in the risk of a peri-procedural serious complication. Although lesion-specific factors such as eccentricity, length, and amount of calcification influenced the complication rate dur-ing angioplasty, hemodynamic intolerance due to the effects of ischemia was often the most important factor influencing the procedural outcome in these high-risk patients. Support measures, such as intra-aortic balloon pump therapy provide a means of substantially improving myocardial tolerance of transient coronary occlusion in these high-risk subsets.

Intra-aortic balloon pump therapy has salutary effects on left ventricular performance and enhances coronary diastolic flow providing hemody-namic stability in high-risk patients. The physiologic effects of intra-aor-tic balloon pump therapy have been reviewed in detail previously. Briefly, intra-aortic balloon pump therapy reduces the afterload against which the left ventricle ejects, significantly reducing myocardial oxygen

Table 5B.1

Cath lab uses of IABP
I.   Elective Revascularization
A. High-risk PTCA
B. Device-specific use (rotational atherectomy)
C. Failed PTCA
II. Emergent
A. Acute MI
1. Prophylactic use following thrombolytic therapy
2. Primary or salvage PTCA
3. Cardiogenic shock
4. Mechanical complications
a. Mitral regurgitation
b. Ventricular septal defect
III. Acute Non-Ischemic Problems
A. Mitral regurgitation
B. Bridge to cardiac transplantation

Key: *PTCA = percutaneous transluminal coronary angioplasty.*

demand. (84, 87, 88) Intra-aortic balloon pump therapy also augments aortic diastolic pressure with a concomitant increase in coronary flow.(13, 14, 37) In animal (32, 91) and clinical studies, (16, 38, 54) use of intra-aortic balloon pump therapy has attenuated or eliminated the effects of ischemia, by the beneficial effect of reducing myocardial oxygen demand. In a recent study by Lazar et al, the effects of intra-aortic balloon pump therapy on indices of myocardial necrosis and function in an animal model were compared to that of percutaneous bypass.(45) Intra-aortic balloon pump therapy resulted in less ischemic damage than percutaneous bypass, and better functional recovery, providing an experimental basis for use of intra-aortic balloon pump therapy in high-risk patients during angioplasty induced ischemia. In patients with severe left ventricular dysfunction, the left ventricle is especially afterload sensitive. Transient occlusion of a coronary artery supplying a critical amount of myocardium will further depress left ventricular systolic function leading to hemodynamic compromise. Intra-aortic balloon pump therapy in this situation may be especially salutary because of its beneficial afterload reducing effects.(32)

Alcan and colleagues were among the first to report on the use of intra-aortic balloon pump therapy in what has been termed a "high-risk" group of patients treated by percutaneous revascularization.(2) Nine patients were treated with balloon angioplasty with a 100% procedural success rate. All of the patients were treated prophylactically with intra-

Table 5B.2

Risk of Percutaneous Transluminal Coronary Angioplasty (PTCA) According to Subgroups*

	No.	Success (%)	MI (%)	EMCABG (%)	Death (%)	Risk Ratio[b]
Total	6500	94	0.5	1.7	0.7	—
Single lesion	2888	93	0.4	2.1	0.6	—
Multiple lesion	3612	95	0.6	1.4	0.8	—
Prior CABG	1225	94	0.6	1.4	0.9	—
"Low-risk"						
Single lesion	1604	88	0.6	2.4	0.3	—
Multiple lesion	1897	96	0.1	1.5	0.2	—
"High-risk"[a]						
Left main	103	92	0.9	1.9	3.9	5.9
Left main equiv[c]	77	95	1.3	6.5	2.6	3.8
EF ≤ 40%	664	93	0.7	2.0	2.7	5.9
Age ≥ 70 (y)	1038	94	0.8	1.3	1.4	2.6
All 3 vessels[d]	305	97	0.6	1.0	1.3	1.9
CATH/PTCA for UA[e]	193	96	1.5	2.0	1.5	2.2
Acute infarction[f]	446	93	—	2.9	8.5	11.2
EF > 30%	383	—	—	—	3.7	5.1
EF < 30%	63	—	—	—	38	52.9
Age < 70 (y)	325	—	—	—	1.5	2.1

[a]Infarct interventions are excluded from "high-risk" subsets except "acute infarction."

[b]Approximate risk relative to all other patients undergoing angioplasty.

[c]From 5000 procedures

[d]From 5568 procedures

[e]From 3197 procedures

[f]From 5000 procedures. Risk ratio is risk of infarct interventions relative to all elective procedures.

Key: *CABG = coronary artery bypass grafting; CATH = catheterization; EF = ejection fraction ; EMCABG = emergency coronary artery bypass surgery; equiv = equivalent; MI = myocardial infarction; UA = unstable angina; — = no data available.*

*Reprinted with permission from Hartzler GO et al. "High-risk" percutaneous transluminal coronary angioplasty. Am J Cardiol 1988;61:33G–37G.

aortic balloon pump therapy. One patient died suddenly 24 hours after the procedure. The authors concluded that intra-aortic balloon pump therapy stabilized hemodynamics, allowing otherwise hemodynamic destabilizing angioplasty to be performed successfully. Since that time, multiple reports of the successful use of angioplasty in high-risk patients with adjunctive balloon pump have been published.(1, 2, 13, 33, 41, 48, 75, 77, 83, 85)

Careful selection of patients considered to be at high risk for coronary angioplasty is essential to the successful completion of the procedure. Of all the currently available support modalities, intra-aortic balloon pump therapy is by far the easiest to use and the most widely accepted (48,49) (Table 5B.3). However, it is limited in augmenting the circulation by its ability to increase cardiac output by approximately 30%, as opposed to femoral bypass where a wide range of cardiac outputs up to 5 L/min can be achieved. It also requires a stable cardiac rhythm. If in our pre-procedural evaluation, a patient is designated as "high risk," we then plan to have a 6 French (Fr) sheath placed in the contralateral femoral artery to maintain arterial access (Figure 5B.1). In addition, a pulmonary artery catheter is placed to measure pulmonary capillary wedge pressure (PCW) during the case. If the PCW is greater than 20 mm Hg, and the area at risk is large, then prophylactic support would be used before the intervention. We would insert a balloon pump if the cardiac output appeared adequate (> 3 L/min), or use peripheral (femoral) bypass support if the cardiac output was already marginal. When the PCW is < 20 mm Hg we use IABP support during the case if hemodynamic compromise or instability arises. Regardless of the support modality chosen, adjunctive hemodynamic support during percutaneous revascularization in patients with LV dysfunction has greatly expanded the management options in these patients.

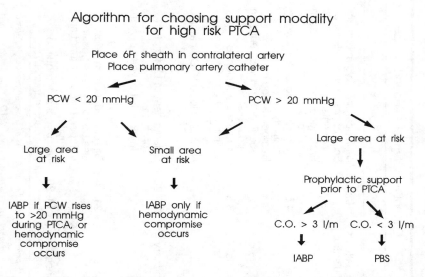

Figure 5B.1. *Schematic diagram depicting an algorithm to aid in choosing a support modality in high-risk patients undergoing angioplasty (PTCA). See text for discussion. IABP = intra-aortic balloon pump; PBS = peripheral (femoral) bypass support; PCW = pulmonary capillary wedge pressure.*

Table 5B.3

Current Percutaneous Support Devices for High-Risk or Complicated Coronary Angioplasty[a]

Device	Size (F)	Advantages	Disadvantages	Applications
Intra-aortic balloon counterpulsation	10.5	↓ Myocardial oxygen demand. Ease of placement in 90% of patients. Prolonged treatment duration possible.	Requires a stable cardiac rhythm and output. 9–43% incidence of vascular complications	Prophlactic placement in selected high-risk patients. Support before CABG with complicated PTCA
Anterograde perfusion	4.5	Improved myocardial oxygen supply. Hemoperfusion or perfluorochemical perfusion possible	Large profile catheter. Ischemia of side branches involving the stenosis. Removal of guidewire needed. Thrombosis risk.	Prolonged balloon inflations expected. Placement before bypass surgery with abrupt closure.
Coronary sinus retroperfusion	8.5	Maintains perfusion to branches compromised by PTCA. No specialized PTCA catheter.	Perfusion improvement documented only in LAD distribution. Incomplete protection from ischemia.	Prolonged balloon inflations in high-risk patients. Investigational.
Cardiopulmonary support	18–20	Independent of LV function or rhythm. ↓ Myocardial oxygen demand.	Complex apparatus and additional arterial and venous access. No improvement of coronary perfusion. 40% vascular complications.	Prophylctic placement in very high-risk patients. Severe hemodynamic compromise after complicated PTCA.
Other devices Hemopump	21	Direct LV decompression. Use up to 14 days possible. Independent of LV function rhythm.	Requires arteriotomy and adequate femoral artery size for placement. Arrhythmogenic LV cannula... Potential for dislodgment from LV.	Investigational
Partial left heart bypass	14–20	No oxygenator required. May decompress LV.	Requires large bore trans-septal cannulation.	Investigational

[a]Reprinted with permission from Lincoff AM, et al. Percutaneous support devices for high risk or complicated coronary angioplasty. J Am Coll Card 1991;17:599–603.

Key: CABG = coronary artery bypass surgery; LAD = left anterior descending artery; LV = left ventricle; PTCA = percutaneous transluminal coronary angioplasty; ↓ = decreased.

Increased use of intra-aortic balloon pump therapy has shifted set-up and management responsibilities from the perfusionists in the operating room to the cardiac catheterization laboratory. Because of the important role of intra-aortic balloon pump therapy as both a prophylactic device during percutaneous revascularization and as a therapeutic device for a variety of patients with cardiac disease it should be an integral part of standard cardiac catheterization equipment. Similarly, because its use is often unanticipated, and is needed urgently, cardiac catheterization laboratory personnel should be thoroughly trained in its set-up and initiation before the arrival of the perfusionist.

Use in Conjunction with Specific Revascularization Devices

Most forms of coronary revascularization currently available involve transient interruption of coronary flow. As such, they all lead to myocardial systolic dysfunction in the regions supplied by the coronary vessel, and hemodynamic compromise depending on the importance of the affected myocardium.(30, 68) In most patients, the myocardial dysfunction recovers quickly after the removal of the device, although sophisticated techniques of measuring myocardial performance indicate persistence of mild abnormalities of diastolic function.(68) Devices that extract or ablate tissue, such as directional coronary atherectomy (DCA), transcutaneous extraction catheter (TEC), and rotational atherectomy (PTCRA) may result in distal embolization, which results in myocardial contractile dysfunction that persists beyond the length of time the device is in the coronary vasculature. For DCA and TEC devices this usually occurs in settings where thrombosis is present such as in the peri-infarction period, in unstable angina, and/or in friable vein grafts. For PTCRA, however, distal embolization of the plaque border may accompany revascularization resulting in a "slow-flow" or "no-reflow" phenomenon in approximately 10% of cases that may persist for several hours after the procedure with significant transient myocardial dysfunction and hemodynamic compromise. Due to this potential problem, intra-aortic balloon pump therapy should always at least be considered as an adjunct to PTCRA in patients with pre-existing left ventricular dysfunction, particularly if the target vessel subtends normally contracting myocardium. Intra-aortic balloon pump therapy in this setting may need to be extended beyond the procedural period for up to several hours until the myocardial dysfunction improves. This is in contradistinction to PTCA when intra-aortic balloon pump therapy can usually be discontinued immediately after a successful procedure.

Use of Intra-aortic Balloon Pump in Failed Elective PTCA

Although PTCA and other revascularization techniques are successful approximately 90% of the time, abrupt vessel closure is a complication in up to 5% of patients.(29) Depending on the contribution of the involved vessel to overall LV performance, abrupt vessel closure may be well tolerated, or may have disastrous hemodynamic effects, including complete hemodynamic collapse. Successful resolution of this problem requires rapid restoration of vessel flow, and often requires hemodynamic support with intra-aortic balloon pump therapy.(8, 11, 29) Murphy et al examined the role of the intra-aortic balloon pump in patients who required emergency bypass surgery after failed PTCA.(56) In patients with ST segment elevation, Q-wave myocardial infarction developed in only 20% of patients (3 of 15) who had intra-aortic balloon pump therapy vs 50% of patients (3 of 6) who did not have balloon pump therapy before emergency bypass. Although this was not statistically significant due to the small sample size, the authors believed intra-aortic balloon pump therapy was clinically important in reducing the effects of ischemia before bypass. Suneja et al reported the use of intra-aortic balloon pump therapy in eight consecutive patients who experienced abrupt vessel closure during PTCA and DCA.(74) In each patient attempts to re-establish flow, including prolonged balloon inflations, were unsuccessful. Intra-aortic balloon pump therapy was then successfully initiated with restoration of coronary flow in all eight patients. Although this represents a small observational study, it suggests that intra-aortic balloon pump therapy may have an important role in this uncommon but significant complication of percutaneous revascularization if restoration of coronary flow cannot be achieved.

Emergent Use during Unstable Angina or Myocardial Infarction

Unstable Angina

Use of IABP Support during PTCA

Patients who present with unstable angina are often successfully treated with antianginal, antiplatelet and anticoagulant therapy. However, a subset of patients with unstable angina are refractory to these therapies and exhibit signs of continued ischemia. Because of the high likelihood of myocardial infarction and increased mortality in this subgroup of patients, invasive management including cardiac catheterization is indicated to define the coronary anatomy.

The mechanism of the beneficial effects of intra-aortic balloon pump therapy in the setting of prolonged ischemia has been evaluated, with somewhat varied results. Williams et al assessed regional myocardial oxygen demand, and coronary blood flow in six patients requiring intra-aortic balloon pump therapy for relief of ischemia.(88) They found a decrease in regional myocardial oxygen demand in five of six patients, whereas regional coronary flow decreased. Fuchs et al studied seven patients requiring intra-aortic balloon pump therapy for unstable angina.(14) In this study the balloon volume was varied and it was found that intra-aortic balloon pump therapy increased flow to the bed fed by collateral vessels or critical stenosis, most likely by augmenting aortic diastolic pressure. Thus, relief of prolonged ischemia by intra-aortic balloon pump therapy probably occurs because of both a reduction in myocardial oxygen demand and an increase in diastolic coronary blood flow.

The clinical utility of intra-aortic balloon pump therapy in unstable angina patients refractory to medical therapy has been reported.(14, 16, 54, 75–77, 88) Szatmary et al used intra-aortic balloon pump therapy in 16 patients with refractory unstable angina. Initiation of balloon pumping alleviated signs of ischemia in all 16 patients, allowing subsequent coronary angioplasty.(76) Angioplasty was successful in 90% of the patients, and there were no complications from the balloon pump itself. Morrison et al reported the use of PTCA in 52 patients with unstable angina, 18 of whom required intra-aortic balloon pump therapy.(54) PTCA was successful in 13 of 18 patients, with no complications from the intra-aortic balloon pump.

In our laboratory, patients with refractory unstable angina are prepared for possible percutaneous revascularization during their initial cardiac catheterization. In addition, a decision is usually made early on whether or not to use intra-aortic balloon pump therapy as an adjunct to the catheterization and/or revascularization procedure. Several factors influence a decision to use intra-aortic balloon pump therapy in this setting. First, any indication that hemodynamic compromise is present, including significant pulmonary edema or hypotension requiring inotropic support, will be an indication that severe LV dysfunction is present and that intra-aortic balloon pump therapy may be required. In these situations the balloon pump would be inserted initially to allow hemodynamic stabilization of the patient and relief of ischemia. Diagnostic cardiac catheterization would then be performed once the intra-aortic balloon pump has been placed and support provided. Second, evidence of progressive ischemia such as further ST segment depression or the appearance or the worsening of ventricular arrhythmias would suggest that intra-aortic balloon pump therapy should be instituted before the diagnostic catheterization. Finally, in the absence of significant LV dysfunction, or worsening ischemia, diagnostic catheterization would be performed first to identify the culprit coronary lesion and the severity of the underlying coronary disease. If a single lesion is present we would proceed with coronary revascularization and use intra-aortic balloon pump therapy only as needed for ischemic compromise during the procedure. On the other hand, if multivessel or left main coronary artery disease were noted, and coronary revascularization was still believed to be the best course of action, an intra-aortic balloon pump would usually be inserted before performing the coronary revascularization.

Use of IABP as a Bridge to Surgery

In the unstable angina patient refractory to medical therapy intra-aortic balloon pump therapy alone may ameliorate ischemia. Since its introduction in 1963, several centers have reported on the beneficial use of intra-aortic balloon pump therapy in patients with prolonged ischemia. Gold et al described the use of intra-aortic balloon pump therapy in 11 patients with angina at rest.(16) Ischemia was alleviated in nine patients, and significantly attenuated in two patients. All 11 patients went on to successful coronary artery bypass surgery.

Stabilization of the patient with intra-aortic balloon pump therapy provides crucial time to allow visualization of the coronary anatomy, as well as thoughtful consideration of the appropriate form of revascularization. We have found this especially useful in a patient with multivessel or left main coronary disease if access to coronary artery bypass grafting is not immediately available. With the patient stabilized by intra-aortic balloon pump therapy, the coronary artery bypass graft operation can be performed under more elective circumstances, and probably at a reduced risk to the patient. A challenging situation arises when an intra-aortic balloon pump is inserted in an unstable angina patient refractory to medical therapy who then stabilizes, but in whom cardiac surgery is not felt to be suitable. As experience with percutaneous revascularization has increased, we have now offered many of these patients angioplasty of the culprit vessel, recognizing that incomplete revascularization will occur. Although this may not be ideal therapy it has allowed effective treatment of many difficult patients.

Acute Myocardial Infarction

There has been significant experience worldwide with the use of intra-aortic balloon pump therapy in acute myocardial infarction. Several studies demonstrated the feasibility of intra-aortic balloon pump therapy in patients with acute myocardial infarction.(9, 12, 17, 59) However, although intra-aortic balloon pump therapy often stabilized hemodynamics in many patients, it had no overall beneficial effect on long-term outcome,(23, 55) probably because the early studies were not accompanied by aggressive coronary revascularization of the underlying problem. Intra-aortic balloon pump therapy was used primarily for mechanical complications of acute myocardial infarction,(17) or for cardiogenic shock. Unfortunately, several studies examining intra-aortic balloon pump therapy for primary therapy of cardiogenic shock complicating myocardial infarction (MI) failed to show any benefit, with survival rates ranging from 5 to 21%.(55) Coronary revascularization concomitant with intra-aortic balloon pump therapy appears to have provided a substantially better outcome for these patients.(6, 15, 42, 46, 47, 53, 71, 86, 89)

Adjunct to Thrombolytic Therapy

The use of intra-aortic balloon pump therapy in the setting of acute myocardial infarction as an adjunct to thrombolytic therapy has been reviewed elsewhere. Briefly, retrospective analysis of data obtained from multiple trials suggested that patients who had intra-aortic balloon pump therapy in the peri-thrombolytic period had a reduced incidence of subsequent coronary reocclusion.(18, 24, 60, 62, 67, 70) Because of the increased morbidity and mortality associated with reocclusion,(61) a prospective trial was undertaken to assess the effects of prophylactic intra-aortic balloon pump therapy on post-thrombolytic coronary artery patency.(63) Ohman and colleagues recently published the results of this trial and showed that prophylactic balloon pumping after thrombolytic therapy was associated with a much lower incidence of reocclusion and reinfarction (10 vs 20%), than patients receiving thrombolytic therapy and standard post-thrombolytic care.(63) In this study the use of the intra-aortic balloon pump did not appear to be associated with an increased incidence of bleeding or other complications. Whether or not large-scale application of intra-aortic balloon pump therapy after successful thrombolytic therapy should be employed remains to be determined. However, its feasibility has been clearly demonstrated by these investigators.

Intra-aortic Balloon Pumping in Conjunction with Primary or Salvage Angioplasty

In the past several years reperfusion therapy for acute myocardial infarction has been expanded to include primary angioplasty.(21, 27, 34, 36, 52, 72, 79, 82) Data supporting its use come from several observational studies (10,36) as well as the PAMI trial, which showed that primary angioplasty was feasible and equally as effective as thrombolytic therapy in patients with acute myocardial infarction.(21) In-hospital recurrent MI and death rates were 10% in the patients who recovered from thrombolytic therapy and 8% in patients treated with PTCA ($P =$ NS).(21) The benefit of PTCA appears to be sustained at 6 months.(73) However, intra-aortic balloon pump therapy was not used as standard adjunct in these studies. It remains to be determined whether prophylactic use of intra-aortic balloon pump therapy in a subset of these patients would be of benefit.

One arm of the PAMI II trial will evaluate prophylactic use of intra-aortic balloon pump therapy following primary PTCA in acute MI.(20) This strategy is based on several observational studies that suggest prophylactic intra-aortic balloon pump therapy may reduce the incidence of post-angioplasty occlusion. First, the study of Ohman et al suggests that intra-aortic balloon pump therapy reduces the incidence of reocclusion following successful thrombolytic therapy.(63) Second, Ishihara et al have shown that intra-aortic balloon pump therapy following successful angioplasty of totally occluded left anterior descending coronary arteries

resulted in a significant decrease in the reocclusion rate (2 vs 18%).(31)
Finally, the data from Stomel et al suggest that intra-aortic balloon pump
therapy in the setting of cardiogenic shock combined with coronary
revascularization results in a substantial improvement in survival.(71)
Although these data are not conclusive, they strongly suggest that adjunctive prophylactic intra-aortic balloon pump therapy may improve the
course of selected patients with acute myocardial infarction undergoing
coronary revascularization. In our laboratory use of intra-aortic balloon
pump therapy is considered in conjunction with primary PTCA of acute
MI if signs of severe LV dysfunction are present, or if the vessel fails to
reperfuse despite repeated or prolonged balloon inflations (Fig. 5B.2).

Use in Cardiogenic Shock

The weight of evidence currently available suggests that intra-aortic balloon pump therapy alone is ineffective in influencing the outcome of
patients with cardiogenic shock. However, beginning in the mid 1980s
several published reports indicated that combined use of coronary revas-

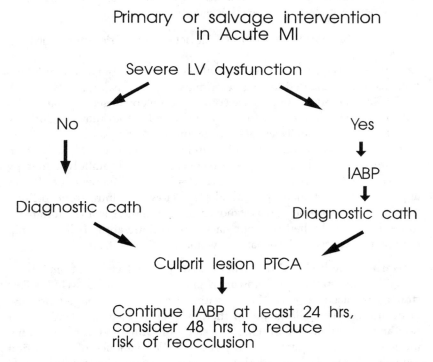

Figure 5B.2. *Schematic diagram showing an approach to patients with acute MI treated
by primary angioplasty or salvage angioplasty following unsuccessful thrombolysis. See text
for details.*

cularization via coronary artery bypass (9, 44, 53, 69) and angioplasty and intra-aortic balloon pump therapy seemed to have a favorable effect on the otherwise dismal course of patients with cardiogenic shock.(3, 25, 46, 47, 55, 58, 71) Although no large randomized trial has been completed to date, several studies have shown that in carefully selected patients the combination of coronary revascularization by angioplasty and intra-aortic balloon pump therapy can be performed safely and with a much more favorable outcome than most previous natural history studies suggest.

Lee et al presented the results of the multicenter registry of angioplasty therapy of cardiogenic shock.(47) This retrospective review of 69 patients treated from 1982 to 1985 showed a substantial benefit of coronary reperfusion with PTCA in this setting (Fig. 5B.3). Patients with successful PTCA had a 69% in-hospital survival, whereas only 20% survived who failed PTCA. Recently, Stomel and colleagues evaluated patients presenting with acute myocardial infarction and cardiogenic shock at community hospitals who were subsequently transferred to a tertiary care hospital.(71) Survival was substantially better in patients receiving reperfusion therapy either with thrombolytics or direct angioplasty (68%) in

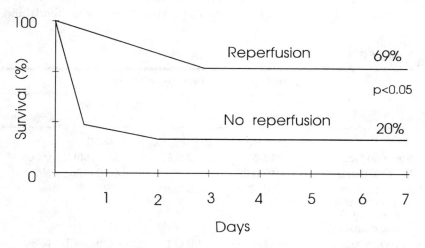

Figure 5B.3. *Graph showing in-hospital survival in patients in the Multicenter Registry for Cardiogenic Shock as a function of coronary reperfusion. Patients who had undergone reperfusion had a substantially higher survival than patients who did not undergo reperfusion. Adapted by permission from Lee L et al. Multicenter registry of angioplasty therapy of cardiogenic shock. Initial and long term survival. J Am Coll Cardiol 1991;17:599–603.*

conjunction with intra-aortic balloon pump therapy vs those who received intra-aortic balloon pump therapy alone (28%) (Table 5B.4). Although this was an observational study and not a randomized trial, it supports the concept that intra-aortic balloon pump therapy alone is not effective as therapy in the setting of an acute myocardial infarction. In conjunction with coronary revascularization intra-aortic balloon pump therapy is a powerful adjunct and appears to substantially alter the poor prognosis of these patients.

Similar to the approach outlined previously for the patient with signs of left ventricular dysfunction and ongoing ischemia, the patient with cardiogenic shock first needs to be stabilized hemodynamically. In our laboratory, this means insertion of an intra-aortic balloon pump before diagnostic cardiac catheterization. Once balloon pumping and diagnostic catheterization have been performed, culprit vessel angioplasty or atherectomy is then performed. Although the exact length of post-procedural intra-aortic balloon pump therapy has not been defined, the study of Ohman et al suggests that a duration of 48 hours should be considered to provide optimal coronary patency and to minimize the incidence of subsequent reocclusion.(63)

The subset of patients with cardiogenic shock from right ventricular infarction deserves special mention. Although shock and right ventricular infarction have been reported in the absence of left ventricular dysfunction, most cases of right ventricular infarction occur in the setting of extensive inferior myocardial infarction. Current treatment includes maximizing right ventricular preload and contractility with fluids and

Table 5B.4

Survival Data in Cardiogenic Shock[a]				
	Thrombolytics	IABP	Thrombolytics plus IABP	P Value
	(n = 13)	(n = 29)	(n = 22)	
Survived No. (%)	3/13 (23)	8/29 (28)	15/22 (68)	0.0049
Medical therapy (%)	1/10 (10)	1/16 (6)	4/10 (40)	N/S
Percutaneous transluminal coronary angioplasty (%)	2/3 (66)	4/5 (80)	3/4 (75)	N/S
Coronary artery bypass graft surgery (%)	0/13	3/8 (38)	8/8 (100)	N/S

Key: N/S = nonsiginificant.

[a]Adapted with permission from Stomel RJ, et al. Treatment Chest strategies for acute myocardial infarction complicated by cardiogenic shock in a community hospital. 1994;105:997–1002.

inotropes.(40) Selective afterload reduction of the right ventricle is an attractive goal but has been difficult to achieve due to inherent difficulties in accessing the pulmonary artery with intra-aortic balloon pump therapy. Pulmonary artery balloon pumps have been tried but require surgical implantation.(51) Vasodilators may have greater effects on systemic vascular resistance than pulmonary vascular resistance, which leads to further hypotension. Insertion of an intra-aortic balloon pump to improve left sided function may have salutary effects in this setting despite the apparent lack of a direct benefit on right ventricular afterload. This may occur via one of several mechanisms. First, intra-aortic balloon pump therapy may augment left ventricular performance, often impaired in right ventricular infarct patients, and indirectly improve right ventricular afterload.(26) Second, in conjunction with pharmacologic or interventional reperfusion, intra-aortic balloon pump therapy may maintain vessel patency and reduce the likelihood of reocclusion. Thus, intra-aortic balloon pump therapy may be useful in the patient with cardiogenic shock from right ventricular infarction.

Use for Mechanical Complications of Myocardial Infarction
Patients with mechanical complications of acute MI often represent the most unstable group of patients with cardiogenic shock complicating acute myocardial infarction. However, with timely intervention these patients may have improved outcomes. Both mitral regurgitation (MR) and ventricular septal defect (VSD) complicating acute MI are responsive to intra-aortic balloon pump therapy. Gold et al have shown that intra-aortic balloon pump therapy in acute VSD reduced the pulmonary to systemic shunt ratio from 5.1 to 4.2 L/min with a concomitant decrease in the pulmonary capillary wedge pressure.(17) Similarly, in acute MR, intra-aortic balloon pump therapy had a beneficial hemodynamic effect with a decrease in the magnitude of the "V" wave, decreased pulmonary capillary wedge pressure, and an increase in cardiac output. Although intra-aortic balloon pump therapy acutely stabilized the hemodynamics in these patients, currently available data suggest that optimal outcomes result when operative repair is performed as rapidly as possible following diagnosis.(17, 43, 64, 80)

The first step in appropriate management of these patients is early recognition of the mechanical problem. This can usually be defined clinically, or with echocardiography. Because of the importance of early intervention, we would not delay bringing the patient to the cardiac catheterization laboratory for non-invasive evaluation. In our catheterization laboratory, an intra-aortic balloon pump is inserted before any diagnostic measures to allow maximal hemodynamic stabilization of the patient. If the mechanical complication has already been recognized or diagnosed, diagnostic cardiac catheterization is performed as soon as feasibly possible after intra-aortic balloon pump therapy is initiated. Unlike management of the patient with cardiogenic shock and acute myocardial infarction defined previously, intra-aortic balloon pump therapy in a patient with acute mitral regurgitation or acute ventricular septal defect is used as a bridge to definitive cardiac surgery and revascularization.

Whether or not a patient with a mechanical complication of acute myocardial infarction should proceed directly to the operating room once the diagnosis has been made or should proceed to the cardiac catheterization laboratory has not been definitively determined. However, several studies suggest that repair of ventricular septal defects or mitral valve replacement for acute mitral regurgitation in the absence of revascularization is associated with a significantly higher mortality than in patients in whom successful revascularization can be performed.(17, 43, 64, 80) Larsson and Svensson described 35 patients with VSD complicating acute MI. (43) Overall operative mortality was 45%. Mortality in patients not receiving coronary artery bypass was 80%. Although these reports represent observations from selected cases, these data support concomitant revascularization during cardiac surgery. At our institution, we take all patients with suspected acute mitral regurgitation or ventricular septal defect complicating acute myocardial infarction to the cardiac catheterization laboratory for intra-aortic balloon pump insertion therapy, and to define their coronary anatomy. Where technically feasible, coronary revascularization accompanies definitive cardiac surgery. In most patients, intra-aortic balloon pump therapy is not needed after definitive repair although some surgeons prefer to use the intra-aortic balloon pump prophylactically during the first 24 hours following surgery.

Use in Severe Non-Ischemic Heart Disease

Use in Severe Non-Ischemic Mitral Regurgitation

Although intra-aortic balloon pump therapy in the cardiac catheterization laboratory is most often used in patients with ischemic heart disease, it is occasionally used in patients with severe non-ischemic mitral regurgitation. This usually arises in the setting of myxomatous mitral valve disease with ruptured chordae tendineae, or in bacterial endocarditis with leaflet perforation. Unlike the patient with mitral regurgitation complicating acute MI, the patient with severe non-ischemic acute MR usually has normal LV function. The afterload reducing effects of intra-aortic balloon pump therapy in this setting are very beneficial and provide substantial improvement in forward cardiac output. Similar to the patient with an ischemic basis for MR, the intra-aortic balloon pump temporizes the clinical situation until definitive mitral valve repair or replacement can be performed.

Use as Bridge to Cardiac Transplantation

Intra-aortic balloon pump therapy may also serve as a temporizing measure in patients with severe class IV congestive heart failure awaiting cardiac transplantation. Prior clinical experience with cardiac transplantation candidates indicated that many patients with an urgent need for transplantation often died while awaiting a donor heart. Because of this problem, many centers have begun using devices, including intra-aortic balloon pump therapy, left ventricular assist devices, (LVAD), and extracorporeal membrane oxygenators (ECMO) to support the patient until a donor heart is available.(36, 65) Although the LVAD and ECMO have been used with success, the intra-aortic balloon pump has been used for up to several weeks and offers greater simplicity of use. Local experience will usually determine the support modality used in these patients.

Complications of Intra-aortic Balloon Pump Therapy

Complications of intra-aortic balloon pump therapy have been reviewed elsewhere. This merits brief attention here because of the frequent use of anticoagulants and thrombolytic agents in patients with acute ischemic heart disease. Several large studies retrospectively evaluated complications in patients treated with intra-aortic balloon pump therapy.(19, 35, 39, 49) Overall, complications occurred in an average of 10% of patients, with irreversible limb ischemia in less than 1% of patients.(19, 35) Patients at higher risk for complications include those with hypertension, diabetes, and female sex (19) as well as pre-existing peripheral vascular disease.(35)

Intra-aortic balloon pumps are now frequently used in patients receiving thrombolytic therapy. During the 1980s, it became clear that the major complication following thrombolytic therapy was bleeding at previous puncture sites, principally those used in cardiac catheterization.(7, 29, 82) Intra-aortic balloon pump therapy theoretically may be associated with higher incidences of vascular complications than diagnostic catheterization alone, because of the increased size of the balloon and the sheaths used. However, currently available data suggest that intra-aortic balloon pump therapy following thrombolytic therapy is not associated with an increased incidence of bleeding.(18, 63, 70) In the randomized IABP study, vascular complications were uncommon in either the catheterized group (2%) and IABP group (5%) with no limb loss. (63) Hemorrhagic complications were also uncommon, and similar rates were observed for both groups. Thus, it would appear that intra-aortic balloon pump therapy per se is not associated with a significant increase in complications over that of cardiac catheterization in this clinical setting.

Many of the previously described studies examined the effects of intra-aortic balloon pumps, often 12 Fr size, before the improvement in balloon size and before more widespread use of percutaneous deployment. The use of smaller balloon shaft sizes, and sheathless insertion (57) may significantly reduce vascular complication rates, and substantially improve the risk to benefit ratio of prophylactic balloon pump use. A major impact in the application on intra-aortic balloon pump therapy could occur if balloon catheter size could be reduced to the 6-Fr or 7-Fr range.

REFERENCES

1. Aguirre FV, et al. Intraaortic balloon pump support during high-risk coronary angioplasty. Cardiology 1994;84:175–186.
2. Alcan KE, Stertzer SH, Wallsh E, DePasquale NP, Bruno MS: The role of intra-aortic balloon counterpulsation in patients undergoing percutaneous transluminal coronary angioplasty Am Heart J 1983;105:527–530.
3. Allen JN, Wewers MD. Acute myocardial infarction with cardiogenic shock during pregnancy: Treatment with intra-aortic balloon counterpulsation. Critical Care Med. 1990;18:888–889.
4. Anwar A, Mooney MR, Stertzer SH, Mooney JF, Shaw RE, Madison JD, VanTassel RA, Murphy MC, Myler RK. Intra-aortic balloon counterpulsation support for elective coronary angioplasty in the setting of poor left ventricular function: A two center experience. J Inv Cardiol 1990;2:175–180.
5. Becker RC. Thrombolytic retreatment with tissue plasminogen activator for threatened reinfarction and thrombotic coronary reocclusion. Clin Cardiol 1994;17:3–13.
6. Bengtson JR, Kaplan AJ, Pieper KS, Wildermann NM, Mark DB, Pryor DB, Phillips HR, Califf RM. Prognosis in cardiogenic shock after acute myocardial infarction in the interventional era. J Am Coll Cardiol 1992;20:1482–1489.
7. Califf RM, Topol EJ, George BS, Boswick JM, Abbottsmith C, Sigmon KN, Candela R, Masek R, Kereiakes D, O'Neill W, Stack RS, Stump D, and the Thrombolysis and Angioplasty in Myocardial Infarction (TAMI) Study Group. Hemorrhagic complications associated with the use of intravenous tissue plasminogen activator in treatment of acute myocardial infarction. Am J Med 1988;85:353–359.
8. Craver JM, Weintraub WS, Jones EL, Guyton RA, Hatcher CR. Emergency coronary artery bypass surgery for failed percutaneous coronary angioplasty. Ann Surg 1992;215:425–433.
9. DeWood MA, Notske RN, Hensley GR, Shields JP, O'Grady WP, Spores J, Goldman M, Ganji JH: Intra-aortic balloon counterpulsation with and without reperfusion for myocardial infarction shock. Circulation 1980;61:1105–1112.
10. Ellis SG, Van de Werf F, Ribeiro-daSilva E, Topol EJ. Present status of rescue coronary angioplasty: current polarization of opinion and randomized trials. J Am Coll Cardiol. 1992;19:681–686.
11. Ferguson TB, Muhlbaier LH, Salai DL, Wechsler AS. Coronary bypass grafting after failed elective and failed emergent percutaneous angioplasty. J Thorac Cardiovasc Surg. 1988;95:761–772.
12. Flaherty JT, Becker LC, Weiss JL, Brinker JA, Bulkley BH, Gerstenblith G, Kallman CH, Weisfeldt ML. Results of a randomized prospective trial of intraaortic balloon counterpulsation and intravenous nitroglycerin in patients with acute myocardial infarction. J Am Coll Cardiol 1985;6:434–446.

13. Flynn MS, Kern MJ, Donohue TJ, Aguirre FV, Bach RG, Caracciolo EA. Alterations of coronary collateral blood flow velocity during intraaortic balloon pump therapy. Am J Cardiol 1993;71:1451–1455.

14. Fuchs RM, Brin KP, Brinker JA, Guzman PA, Heuser RR, Yin FCP. Augmentation of regional coronary blood flow by intra-aortic balloon counterpulsation in patients with unstable angina. Circulation 1983;68:117–123.

15. Gacioch GM, et al. Cardiogenic shock complicating acute myocardial infarction: The use of coronary angioplasty and the integration of the new support devices into patient management. J Am Coll Cardiol 1992;19:647–653.

16. Gold HK, Leinbach RC, Sanders CA, Buckley MJ, Munth ED, Austen WG. Intraaortic balloon pump therapy for control of recurrent myocardial ischemia. Circulation 1973;47:1197–1203.

17. Gold HK, Leinbach RC, Sanders CA, Buckley MJ, Munth ED, Austen WG. Intraaortic balloon pump therapy for ventricular septal defect or mitral regurgitation complicating acute myocardial infarction. Circulation 1973;47:1191–1196.

18. Goodwin M, et al. Safety of intraaortic balloon counterpulsation in patients with acute myocardial infarction receiving streptokinase intravenously. Am J Cardiol 1989;64:937–938.

19. Gottlieb SO, et al. Identification of patients at high risk for complications of intraaortic balloon counterpulsation: A multivariate risk factor analysis. Am J Cardiol 1984;53:1135–1139.

20. Griffin J, et al. A prospective, randomized trial evaluation of the prophylactic use of balloon pumping in high risk myocardial infarction patients: PAMI 2. JACC 1995;25:86A.

21. Grines CL, Browne KR, Marco, et al. A comparison of primary angioplasty with thrombolytic therapy for acute myocardial infarction. N Engl J Med 1993;328:673–679.

22. Gruppo Italiano per lo Studio della Streptochinasi nell'Infarto Miocardico (GISSI). Effectiveness of intravenous thrombolytic treatment in acute myocardial infarction. Lancet 1988;I:397–401.

23. Gunnar RM. Cardiogenic shock complicating acute myocardial infarction. Circulation. 1988;78:1508–1510.

24. Gurbel PA, Anderson RD, MacCord CS, Scott H, Komjathy SF, Poulton J, Stafford JL, Godard J. Arterial diastolic pressure augmentation by intra-aortic balloon counterpulsation enhances the onset of coronary artery reperfusion by thrombolytic therapy. Circulation. 1994;89:361–365.

25. Hands ME, et al. The in-hospital development of cardiogenic shock after myocardial infarction: Incidence, predictors of occurrence outcome and prognostic factors. J Am Coll Cardiol 1989;14:40–46.

26. Hansan RIR, Deiranyia AK, Yonan NA. Effect of intra-aortic balloon counterpulsation on right-left shunt following right ventricular infarction. Internat J Cardiol 1991;33:439–442.

27. Hargreaves M, Channon K, Ormerod O. Emergency percutaneous transluminal coronary angioplasty (PTCA) for intractable ventricular arrhythmias associated with acute anterior myocardial infarction. Br Heart J. 1993;70:485–486.

28. Hartzler GO, Rutherford BD, McConahay DR, Johnson WL, Giorgi LV: "High-risk" percutaneous transluminal coronary angioplasty. Am J Cardiol 1988;61:33G–37G.

29. Holmes DR Jr. Complications. In: Vliestra RE, Holmes DR Jr, eds. PTCA: Percutaneous Transluminal coronary angioplasty. Philadelphia: FA Davis; 1987; p 145.

30. Ishihara M, Sato H, Tateishi H, Kawagoe T, Muraoka Y, Yoshimura M. Effects of intraaortic balloon pump therapy on coronary hemodynamics after coronary angioplasty in patients with acute myocardial infarction. Am Heart J. 1992;124:1133–1138.

31. Ishihara M, Sato H, Tateishi H, Uchida T, Dote K. Intraaortic balloon pump therapy as the postangioplasty strategy in acute myocardial infarction. Am H J 1991;122:385–389.

32. Jie C, Yisheng J, Fuzen F, Jun Z, Min Z, Weilian Z, Lifan Z. The effect of IABP ventricular contractility of the normal and ischemic canine heart assessed in situ by T–Emax. Adv Exp Med Biol 1989;248:517–525.

33. Kahn JK, Rutherford BD, McConahay DR, Johnson WL, Giorgi LV, Hartzler GO. Supported "high risk" coronary angioplasty using intraaortic balloon pump counterpulsation. J Am Coll Cardiol 1990;15:1151–1155.

34. Kahn JK, et al. Results of primary angioplasty for acute myocardial infarction in patients with multivessel coronary artery disease. J Am Coll Cardiol 1990;16:1089–1096.

35. Kantrowitz A, Wasfie T, Freed PS, Rubenfire M, Wajszczuk W, Schork MA. Intraaortic balloon pump therapy 1967 through 1982: Analysis of complications in 733 patients. Am J Cardiol. 1986;57:976–983.

36. Kaye MP. The registry of the international society for heart and lung transplantation: Tenth official report–1993. Registry 1993;12:541–548.

37. Kern MJ, Aguirre FV, Bach R, Donohue T, Siegel R, Segal J. Augmentation of coronary blood flow by intra-aortic balloon pumping in patients after coronary angioplasty. Circulation. 1993;87:500–511.

38. Kern MJ, et al. Enhanced coronary blood flow velocity during intraaortic balloon counterpulsation in critically ill patients. J Am Coll Cardiol 1993;21: 359–368.

39. Kern MJ. Intra-aortic balloon counterpulsation. Cor Artery Dis 1991;2: 649–660.

40. Kinch JW, Ryan TJ. Current Concepts: Right ventricular infarction. N Engl J Med 1994;330:1211–1217.

41. Kreidieh I, Davies DW, Lim R, Nathan AW, Dymond DS, Banim SO. High-risk coronary angioplasty with elective intra-aortic balloon pump support. Inter J Cardiol 1992;35:147–152.

42. Kuchar DL, Campbell TJ, O'Rourke MF. Long-term survival after counterpulsation for medically refractory heart failure complicating myocardial infarction and cardiac surgery. Eur Heart J 1987;8:490–502.

43. Larsson S, Svensson S. Management of postinfarction ventricular septal rupture. Thorac Cardivasc Surg. 1987;35:180–184.

44. Lazar HL, Yang XM, Rivers S, Treanor P, Shemin RJ. Role of percutaneous bypass in reducing infarct size after revascularization for acute coronary insufficiency. Circulation. 1991;84(suppl lll):416–421.

45. Lazar HL,Yang XM, Rivers S, Treanor P, Bernard S, Shemin R. Retroperfusion and balloon support to improve coronary revascularization. J Cardiovasc Surg. 1992;33:538–544.

46. Lee L, Bates E, Pitt B, Walton J, Laufer N, O'Neill WW: Percutaneous transluminal coronary angioplasty improves survival in acute myocardial infarction complicated by cardiogenic shock. Circulation 1988;78:1345–1351.

47. Lee L, Erbel R, Brown TM, Laufer N, Meyer J, O'Neill WW. Multicenter registry of angioplasty therapy of cardiogenic shock. Initial and long term survival. J Am Coll Cardiol 1991;17:599–603.

48. Lincoff AM, Popma JJ, Ellis SG, Vogel RA, Topol EJ. Percutaneous support devices for high risk or complicated coronary angioplasty. J Am Coll Cardiol 1991;17:770–780.

49. Maccioli GA, Lucas WJ, Norfleet EA. The intra-aortic balloon pump: A review. J Cardiothorac Anesthesiol 1988;2:365–373.

50. Maiello L, Colombo A, Gianrossi R, Almagor Y, Finci L. Survival after percutaneous transluminal coronary angioplasty in patients with severe left ventricular dysfunction. Chest. 1994;105:733–740.

51. Miller DC, Moreno-Cabral RJ, Stinson EB, Shinn JA, Shumway NE. Pulmonary artery balloon counterpulsation for acute right ventricular failure. J Thorac Cardiovasc Surg 1980;80:760–763.

52. Misinski M. Role of conventional management and alternative therapies in limiting infarct size in acute myocardial infarction. Heart Lung. 1987;16:746–755.

53. Moosvi AR, Khaja F, Villanueva L, Gheorghiade M, Douthat L, Goldstein S. Early revascularization improves survival in cardiogenic shock complicating acute myocardial infarction. J Am Coll Cardiol 1992;19:907–914.

54. Morrison DA, Barbierre C, Cohan A, Olsen MA, Stovall R, Wolff D. Percutaneous transluminal coronary angioplasty for rest angina pectoris requiring intravenous nitroglycerin and intraaortic balloon counterpulsation. Am J Cardiol 1990;66:168–171.

55. Mueller HS. Role of intra-aortic counterpulsation in cardiogenic shock and acute myocardial infarction. Cardiology. 1994;84:168–174.

56. Murphy DA, et al. Surgical management of acute myocardial ischemia following percutaneous transluminal coronary angioplasty. J Thorac Cardiovasc Surg 1984;87:332–339.

57. Nash IS, Lorell BH, Fishman RF, Baim DS, Donahue C, Diver DJ. A new technique for sheathless percutaneous intraaortic balloon catheter insertion. Cathet Cardiovasc Diagn 1991;23:57–60.

58. O'Neill WW. Angioplasty therapy of cardiogenic shock: Are randomized trials necessary? J Am Coll Cardiol 1992;19:915–917.

59. O'Rourke MF, Norris RM, Campbell TJ, Chang VP, Sammel NL. Randomized controlled trial of intraaortic balloon counterpulsation in early myocardial infarction with acute heart failure. Am J Cardiol 1981;47:815–820.

60. Ohman EM et al and the Thrombolysis and Angioplasty in Myocardial Infarction (TAMI) Study Group. The use of intraaortic balloon pump therapy as an adjunct to reperfusion therapy in acute myocardial infarction. Am Heart J 1991;121:895–901.

61. Ohman EM, et al. Consequences of reocclusion after successful reperfusion therapy in acute myocardial infarction: TAMI Study Group. Circulation. 1990;82:781–791.

62. Ohman EM et al and the TAMI Study Group. Aortic counterpulsation with thrombolysis for myocardial infarction: Salutary effect on reocclusion on the infarct related artery. J Am Coll Cardiol 1992;19(suppl A):381A.

63. Ohman EM et al for the Randomized IABP Study Group. Use of aortic counterpulsation to improve sustained coronary artery patency during acute myocardial infarction. Circulation 1994;90:792–799.

64. Pappas PJ, Cernaianu AC, Baldino WA, Cilley JH, DelRossi AJ. Ventricular free-wall rupture after myocardial infarction: Treatment and outcome. Chest 1991;99:892–895.

65. Pennington DG, Termuhlen DF. Mechanical circulatory support: Device selection. In: Emery RW, Pritzker MR, Eales F, eds. Cardiothoracic Transplantation II. Cardiac Surgery: State of art reviews. Vol. 3, no. 3. Philadelphia: Hanley and Belfus; 1989.

66. Phillips SJ, et al. Benefits of combined balloon pumping and percutaneous cardiopulmonary bypass. Ann Thorac Surg 1992;54:908–910.

67. Prewitt RM, Gu S, Schick U, Ducas J. Intraaortic balloon counterpulsation enhances coronary thrombolysis induced by intravenous administration of a thrombolytic agent. J Am Coll Cardiol 1994;23:794–798.

68. Serruys PW, et al. Left ventricular performance, regional blood flow, wall motion and lactate metabolism during transluminal angioplasty. Circulation 1984;70:25–36.

69. Sharp TG, Kesler KA. Surgical myocardial revascularization after acute infarction. Chest. 1993;104:1063–1069.

70. Silverman AJ, Wetmore RW. Intraaortic balloon pump and thrombolysis in AMI. Am Heart J 1992;123:1720.

71. Stomel RJ, Rasak M, Bates ER. Treatment strategies for acute myocardial infarction complicated by cardiogenic shock in a community hospital. Chest. 1994;105:997–1002.

72. Stone GW, et al. Direct coronary angioplasty in acute myocardial infarction: outcome in patients with single vessel disease. J Am Coll Cardiol 1990;15:534–543.

73. Stone, GW, et al. Predictors of in-hospital and 6-month outcome after acute myocardial infarction in the reperfusion era: The primary angioplasty in myocardial infarction (PAMI) trial. JACC 1995;25:370–377.

74. Suneja R, McBarron Hodgson J. Use of intraaortic balloon counterpulsation for treatment of recurrent acute closure after coronary angioplasty. Am Heart J 1993;125:530–532.

75. Szatmary LJ, Marco J, Fajadet J, Caster L, Carrie D. Intraaortic balloon counterpulsation and coronary angioplasty in high risk coronary heart patients. Acta Medica Hungarica. 1987;44:189–200.

76. Szatmary LJ, Marco J, Fajadet J, Caster L. The combined use of diastolic counterpulsation and coronary dilation in unstable angina due to multivessel disease under unstable hemodynamic conditions. Inter J Cardiol 1988; 19:59–66.

77. Szatmary LJ, Marco J. Haemodynamic and antiischaemic protective effects of intra-aortic balloon counterpulsation in high risk coronary heart patients undergoing percutaneous transluminal coronary angioplasty. Cor Vasa 1987;29:183–191.

78. Talley JD, Jones EL, Weintraub WS, King SB. Coronary artery bypass surgery after failed elective percutaneous transluminal coronary angioplasty. Circulation. 1989;79:I126–I133.

79. The TIMI Study Group. The Thrombolysis in Myocardial Infarction (TIMI) trial. N Engl J Med 1985;312:932–936.

80. Topaz D, Taylor AL. Interventricular septal rupture complicating acute myocardial infarction: From pathophysiologic features to the role of invasive and noninvasive diagnostic modalities in current management. Am J Med 1992;93:683–688.

81. Topol EJ, et al. Confronting the issues of patients safety and investigator conflict of interest in an international clinical trial of myocardial reperfusion. J Am Coll Cardiol 1992;1:1123–1128.

82. Topol EJ et al and the Thrombolysis and Angioplasty in Myocardial Infarction (TAMI) Study Group. A randomized trial of late reperfusion therapy for acute myocardial infarction. Circulation. 1992;85:2090–2099.

83. Ueda O, Kohchi K, Koga N. Percutaneous transluminal coronary angioplasty with cardiopulmonary bypass for stenosis of the most proximal part of the left anterior descending coronary artery. Br Heart J 1990;63:178–179.

84. Urschel CW, Eber L, Forrester J, Matloff J, Carpenter R, Sonnenblick E. Alteration of mechanical performance of the ventricle by intraaortic balloon counterpulsation. Am J Cardiol 1970;25:546–551.

85. Voudris V, Marco J, Morice MC, Fajadet J, Royer T. "High-risk" percutaneous transluminal coronary angioplasty with preventive intra-aortic balloon counterpulsation. Cathet Cardiovasc Diagn 1990;19:160–164.

86. Waksman R, Weiss AT, Gotsman MS, Hasin Y. Intra-aortic balloon counterpulsation improves survival in cardiogenic shock complicating acute myocardial infarction. Eur Heart J 1993;14:71–74.

87. Weber KT, Janicki JS. Intraaortic balloon counterpulsation. A review of physiological principles, clinical results, and device safety. Ann Thorac Surg 1974;17:603–636.

88. Williams DO, Korr KS, Gewirtz H, Most AS. The effect of intraaortic balloon counterpulsation on regional myocardial blood flow and oxygen consumption in the presence of coronary artery stenosis in patients with unstable angina. Circulation 1982;66:593–597.

89. Woronow DI. Community hospital implementation of intraaortic balloon pump therapy for complicated myocardial infarction. Maryland Med J 1992;41:227–229.

90. Zalewski A, Savage M, Goldberg S. Protection of the ischemic myocardium during percutaneous transluminal coronary angioplasty. Am J Cardiol 1988;61:54G–60G.

91. Zobel G, Dacar D, Kuttnig M, Rodl S, Rigler B. Mechanical support of the left ventricle in ischemia induced left ventricular failure: An experimental study. Inter J Artif Organs. 1992;15:114–119.

5

PART C

Use of the Intra-aortic Balloon Pump for Post-Cardiotomy Support

Mark P. Anstadt ▪ Mark F. Newman

Introduction

It is estimated that over 250,000 open heart procedures are performed each year in the United States (1) and that approximately 600,000 occur worldwide.(2) These procedures are now considered relatively routine and carry a relatively low mortality (1–3%). However, as many as 5 to 12% of patients suffer post-cardiotomy cardiogenic shock or "pump failure." The associated mortality approaches 50% and emphasizes the challenges created by this patient population. Less than 30 years ago patients who experienced cardiogenic shock, even for a few hours, were uniformly anticipated to perish, hence the term, "irreversible shock".(3) This concept originated before clinically feasible methods of assisted circulation became available. The IABP has since offered a unique, life-saving therapy for patients in cardiogenic shock. Early experience using IABP support in the treatment of cardiogenic shock demonstrated its potential to improve myocardial function while reducing the myocardium's energy requirements. In this manner, the IABP could restore organ perfusion without further compromising the myocardium, thereby, ameliorating the otherwise irreversible pathophysiology of post-cardiotomy cardiogenic shock.

Many of the physiologic principles that are fundamental to IABP effectiveness for post-cardiotomy support were realized before the device's inception. As early as 1953, the Kantrowitz brothers demonstrated a concept, which later proved fundamental to the IABPs efficacy. Their novel experimental work demonstrated that the delayed arrival of systolic pressure to the coronary circulation by an interposed rubber conduit improved myocardial perfusion. This phenomenon, termed diastolic augmentation, was subsequently exploited by the technique of diastolic aorta compression using a surgically transferred hemidiaphragm.(4) Harken (5) postulated that aspiration of arterial blood during systole, and reinfusion during diastole, could diminish cardiac work without compromising perfusion. Later, a device developed by Clauss and associates (6) achieved "diastolic counterpulsation" by withdrawing and infusing blood via two femoral artery cannulas. The most practical means of achieving diastolic augmentation was later reported by both Clauss (7) and Moulopoulos (8) while working in independent laboratories. Both investigators demonstrated that balloons positioned in the central aorta could augment diastolic pressure if inflated and deflated synchronous to the cardiac cycle. This simple, yet ingenious method of intravascular volume displacement has evolved into the modern intra-aortic balloon pump (IABP) (Fig. 5C.1).

Physiologic Considerations

Post-cardiotomy cardiogenic shock can result from either primary myocardial pump failure or peripheral vascular collapse. Most commonly, the underlying problem necessitating IABP therapy is pump failure secondary to myocardial ischemia, cardiomyopathy or valvular disease.

The IABP is typically employed on a temporary basis with two primary therapeutic goals: improve organ perfusion to preserve vital function and reduce cardiac work to interrupt progressive myocardial injury. By successfully reversing the pathophysiologic consequences of cardiogenic shock, the IABP facilitates separation from cardiopulmonary bypass and improvement in myocardial function. Successful separation from cardiopulmonary bypass is predicated on a fundamental understanding that normal myocardial function requires that the right and left ventricles operate as two pumps in series. The left ventricle will most commonly require assistance when significant cardiac decompensation occurs. For this reason, most cardiovascular compensatory mechanisms have been characterized for the left ventricle (LV) and the systemic circulation. However, these principles can also be applied to the right ventricle (RV) and pulmonary circulation. Because the right and left ventricles function in series, their performance must remain balanced over a wide range of physiologic states. These conditions are satisfied by the Frank-Starling law of the heart. Normally, each ventricle operates within a relatively narrow range of end-diastolic volumes (EDV) or preloads. Changes in preload occur with fluctuations in venous return, and are accommodated by variations in ventricular geometry. The degree of ventricular distention, in turn, alters the alignment of actin and myosin filaments, thereby modulating myocardial contractility. In this manner, the Frank-Starling relationship

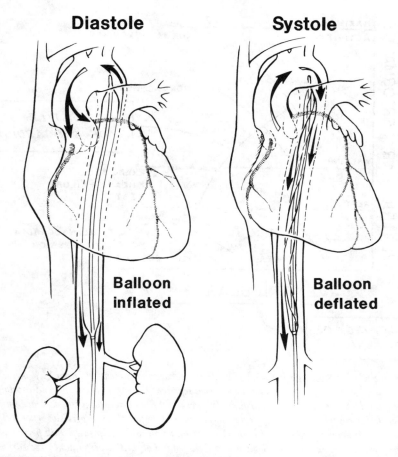

Diastole   **Systole**

Balloon inflated   **Balloon deflated**

Figure 5C.1. *Schematic representation of a properly positioned intra-aortic balloon pump. Arrows indicate direction of blood volume displacement. During diastole, balloon inflation displaces blood, which augments coronary perfusion pressure. During systole, balloon deflation reduces resistance to forward flow. Reprinted with permission from Anstadt MP. Acquired cardiac conditions: Cardiac assist devices and the artificial heart. In: Sabiston DC, Lyerly HK, eds. Essentials of Surgery. Philadelphia: WB Saunders; 1994.*

accounts for most normal changes in cardiac output and accounts for maintaining balanced flow between the right and left ventricles.

The Frank-Starling relationship is best illustrated by ventricular pressure-volume curves. "Starling curves" (Fig. 5C.2) depict changes in myocardial performance that result from physiologic alterations in preload and contractility. Load-dependent adjustments in performance help maintain ventricular output within an optimal range. When this mechanism is not sufficient to meet increased physiologic demands, other factors (eg,

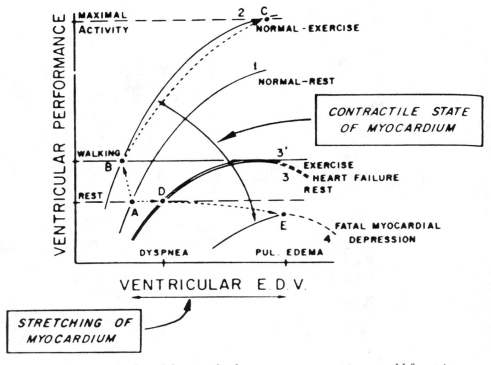

Figure 5C.2. *Starling's left ventricular function curves, representing normal left ventric-ular function at rest and exercise (upper curves represent increased ventricular end-diastolic volume). Depressed left ventricular function may result from myocardial ischemia or infarc-tion (lower curves show varying degrees of myocardial dysfunction). Progressive myocardial dysfunction may eventually lead to fatal myocardial depression. Reprinted with permission from Braunwald E, Ross J Jr, Sonnenblick EH. Control of cardiac performance and cardiac output: A Synthesis. In Braunwald E, Ross J, Sonnenblick EH, eds. Mechanisms of Contraction of the Normal and Failing Heart. Boston: Little Brown and Co; 1968.*

increased heart rate, endogenous catecholamines) can independently influence the heart's contractile state and "shift" the Starling curve upward. On the other hand, myocardial ischemia depresses cardiac func-tion causing a "downward shift" in the Starling curve. Consequently, the ischemic heart contracts less vigorously for any given EDV and is less responsive to further increases in preload.

In the setting of myocardial ischemia, increased EDV may initially com-pensate for decreased contractility. However, these salutary effects become less adequate as cardiac pathology worsens. If LV distention con-tinues to progress, the optimal wall tension for actin and myosin interac-tions is surpassed, which further impairs contractile function. Reduced ventricular compliance is exhibited by disproportionate elevations in end-diastolic pressure with further increases in preload. Continued cardiac injury eventually results in virtual loss of the compensatory response as the heart dilates. The deleterious effects of ventricular distention are based on Laplace's law.

$$T = P \times R/h$$

where T = ventricular wall tension, P = intraventricular pressure, R = intracavitary radius, and h = ventricular wall thickness. Ventricular dilatation increases wall tension, creating an even greater demand for effective ventricular contraction. The cycle then set in motion places increasing stress on an already compromised heart. Cardiac output further declines, exacerbating the ischemic process that initiated these events. Brief periods of ventricular distention, in and of itself, can result in irreversible myocardial damage.

The typical physiologic response to low cardiac output is largely mediated by the sympathetic nervous system. However, this places increased demands on the failing heart. Endogenous catecholamines directly stimulate the heart to contract more vigorously and also increase peripheral vascular resistance. It has long been known that increases in afterload (pressure work) are significantly more costly in terms of myocardial oxygen consumption than increases in cardiac output (volume work).[9] Factors such as heart rate and temperature also affect myocardial oxygen demand, but to a lesser degree. Therefore, the primary hemodynamic determinants of myocardial oxygen consumption are best delineated by the time-tension index (TTI), Figure 5C.3. In contrast, the diastolic pressure time index (DPTI) represents the driving force for coronary blood flow, and serves as a measure of myocardial oxygen delivery. The balance between myocardial oxygen supply and demand, or the DPTI/TTI ratio, is termed the "endocardial viability ratio" because of the endocardium's marked susceptibility to ischemia.

Therapeutic Approach to Post-Cardiotomy Pump Failure

Collectively, the cardiac surgeon, anesthesiologist, and perfusionist use the previously described principles to manipulate and optimize the cardiovascular system when separating patients from cardiopulmonary bypass. The following guidelines represent general strategies undertaken at Duke University Medical Center. Separation from bypass at almost all institutions represents the initial optimization of heart rate and preload. Adequate heart rate, greater than 70 beats per minute, is achieved either from sinus rhythm, atrial or atrioventricular pacing, followed by the optimization of preload based on prebypass filling pressure. This provides the surgeon and anesthesiologist an indication of ventricular function at low to moderate filling pressures. Based on this initial information further

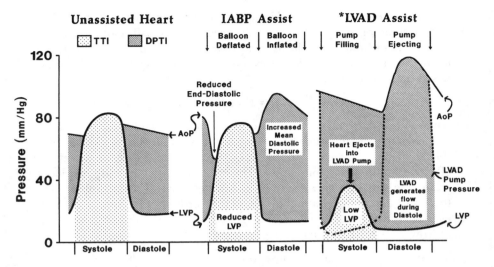

Figure 5C.3. *Hemodynamic determinants of myocardial oxygen demand (time tension index [TTI]) and delivery (diastolic pressure time index [DPTI]) are illustrated for the failing unassisted heart, and during intra-aortic balloon pump (IABP) and left ventricular assist device (LVAD) therapies. AoP = aortic pressure, LVP = left ventricular pressure. (*Hemodynamic alterations representative for synchronized LVAD counterpulsation.) Reprinted with permission from Anstadt MP. Acquired cardiac conditions: Cardiac assist devices and the artificial heart. In: Sabiston DC, Lyerly HK, eds. Essentials of Surgery. Philadelphia: WB Saunders; 1994.*

assessment is made to determine the need for inotropes. Periods of significant hypotension with elevated filling pressures should be avoided to minimize the potential for myocardial ischemia. Although small doses of neosynephrine, calcium, or epinephrine can be used to bide time for initiating other therapies, an early decision to return to bypass and rest the heart remains a more conservative and informed approach. Subsequent selections of inotropic therapy relate to left ventricular function as well as calculated systemic vascular resistance. Transesophageal echocardiography (TEE) has been shown to provide additional valuable information when weaning from bypass. It has been demonstrated that early utilization of TEE can alter inotrope selection and improve the decision for other interventions in 10 to 15% of cases.(10)

The first line inotropic agent at Duke University Medical Center is generally dopamine at 5 to 7 μg/kg/min. Dopamine is used because of its variable beta to alpha response over differing dose ranges. The addition of nitroglycerin or nipride frequently allows one to achieve the desired level of inotropy and chronotropy with varying degrees of systemic vascular resistance. Dobutamine represents another option however, it limits the ability to independently control inotropy and systemic vascular resistance in the immediate postbypass period. The selected therapeutic approach must be succeeded by an adequate time interval to evaluate the patient's functional response just as with the initial separation from bypass.

Determining the need for a second line inotropic agent relates similarly to the assessment of heart rate, preload, cardiac index and systemic vascular resistance (SVR). An algorithm that leads to appropriate decision making is outlined in Figure 5C.4. The general goal of this cascade is to achieve the necessary pressure and flow to provide adequate end-organ perfusion. Once it becomes evident that the underlying problem is pump failure, improved myocardial performance should be accomplished in a sequence that least increases myocardial oxygen demand as outlined in the following text:

1. Increase cardiac output (CO) by optimizing heart rate (70 to 90 bpm) and preload (left atrial pressure or pulmonary capillary wedge pressure of 10 to 15 mm Hg).
2. If CO remains low ($<$ 1.8 to 2.0 L/min/m^2):
   a. Institute vasodilators to decrease SVR (if elevated) and reoptimize preload as required following this intervention.
   b. Add or increase inotropic support if SVR is low or normal or if patient becomes hypotensive with reduced CO.
3. Employ a vasoconstrictor if the SVR is low in the setting of a normal to elevated CO and relative hypotension. (Note: prolonged use of vasoconstrictors may decrease renal perfusion and, thereby, compromise renal function.)
4. Cardiac output and hemodynamic parameters should be reassessed, and appropriate pharmacologic agents (additional inotropes and/or vasodilators) instituted as indicated by revisiting the algorithm from Figure 5C.4.

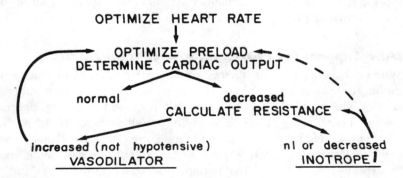

Figure 5C.4. *Schematic algorithm for the treatment of low cardiac output syndrome. Reprinted with permission from Reves JG. Vasoactive drugs and when to use them. In: Stephen Thomas, ed. Manual of Cardiac Anesthesia. Churchill Livingstone, NY; 1984.*

Secondary inotropic agents are typically used before consideration of mechanical support. Epinephrine, milrinone, or the synergistic combination of these agents,(11) are generally used in accordance with the hemodynamic milieu. If available, TEE may serve to guide therapy at this point. In particular, TEE can differentiate global and regional LV dysfunction as well as assess any relevant concerns of valvular function. Significant regional wall motion abnormalities may indicate ongoing ischemia, infarction or stunning. If this situation is not felt related to a technical or metabolic problem, further inotropic support may only exacerbate the problem. Global dysfunction and/or moderate degrees of regional stunning may respond favorably to increased inotropic support but only at the expense of increased myocardial oxygen demands.

Optimal medical management of severe left ventricular power failure should be directed towards improving the unfavorable balance between myocardial oxygen supply and demand. Beta-blocking agents decrease myocardial oxygen demand, but may decrease ventricular performance, which further compromises end-organ perfusion.(12) Patients in cardiogenic shock generally require high doses of inotropic agents, which maintain organ perfusion by increasing myocardial contractility.(13) These agents cause a concomitant increase in myocardial oxygen consumption and frequently exacerbate myocardial ischemia. Afterload reducing agents lessen these negative effects by reducing ventricular work, but caution must be exercised to avoid jeopardizing coronary perfusion. Ideally, any potential underlying pathology amenable to further surgical repair should be ruled out and corrected if possible. If these measures fail to adequately restore hemodynamics and tissue perfusion as evidenced by urine output < 0.5 cc/kg/h, cardiac index > 2.0 L/min/m^2, and the presence of progressive acidosis, then mechanical circulatory support should be strongly considered. Other clinical scenarios in which the threshold for mechanical circulatory support may supersede more routine pharmacologic regimens are listed in Table 5C.1.

IABP Support for Post-Cardiotomy Pump Failure

When circulatory support is necessary, the IABP is generally considered the most appropriate initial therapy. In general, most patients suffering cardiogenic shock who do not adequately respond to maximal pharmacologic measures are considered potential candidates for IABP support (Table 5C.2). However, the appropriate regimen of pharmacologic therapy before initiating IABP support remains controversial. Some argue that earlier institution of IABP therapy may decrease the risk of further end-organ damage that frequently complicates the prolonged use of high dose inotropic agents. These unresolved issues, along with the fact that some of the indications for IABP support remain controversial, explain

Table 5C.1

Criteria That May Lower the Threshold for Post-Cardiotomy IABP Support

Poor revascularization
New or ongoing ischemia
Diffuse CAD
Technical problems with grafts
Poor protection
Long ischemic and/or CPB time
Repeated evidence of electrical activity during cross-clamp
Preoperative or prebypass IABP insertion

Key: *CAD = coronary artery disease; CPB = cardiopulmonary bypass; IABP = intra-aortic balloon pump.*

Table 5C.2

General Criteria for IABP Support Following Cardiac Surgery

Inability to separate from CPB despite multiple interventions after 30 min
Inadequate hemodynamics despite maximal inotropic support including:
Persistent hypotension (systolic blood pressure < 70 mm Hg)
Low cardiac index (<2.0 L/min/m²)
Elevated left atrial pressure (>20 mm Hg)
High peripheral vascular resistance (>2500 dynes/sec/cm⁻⁵)
Requirement of inotropic agents at deleterious levels
Persistent malignant ventricular arrhythmias

Key: *CPB = cardiopulmonary bypass.*

the apparent variations in IABP utilization among reporting institutions (Table 5C.3).(14) In any event, IABP therapy offers the failing heart a mechanical advantage that no pharmaceutical interventions can provide. Furthermore, IABP insertion requires minimal technical skill and, if necessary, can be accomplished at the bedside.

The IABP is not a true blood pump, but improves the balance between myocardial oxygen supply and demand by displacing intravascular volume (see Fig. 5C.1). The device's balloon occupies (inflation) and vacates (deflation) space within the central aorta during diastole and systole, respectively. Two favorable hemodynamic changes result (15, 16) (see Fig. 5C.3). First, mean diastolic blood pressure increases due to aortic volume displacement during balloon inflation. Second, afterload is reduced by the aortic vacancy caused by balloon deflation just before ventricular emptying. Diastolic augmentation, the term adopted to describe these hemodynamic alterations, highlights the increase in coro-

Table 5C.3

	Adult Cardiac Procedures N	Frequency of IABP Insertion		30-day mortality (%)	2-year survival (%)
		No.	%		
Washington University	6877	432	6.3	34	56
Duke University	3297	90	3.0	40	42
Texas Heart Institute and Baylor College of Medicine	2813	322	11.4	48	ND
St. Louis University	6856	473	6.9	42	49

Modern Survival Results for Postcardiotomy IABP

Key: ND = no data available.

nary perfusion pressure that can alleviate myocardial ischemia.(17,18) However, it should be emphasized that afterload reduction is the most beneficial effect of the IABP on the failing heart.(19, 20) When IABP support is insufficient, ventricular assist devices can maximize afterload reduction and diastolic augmentation if properly synchronized with the cardiac cycle (see Fig. 5C.3).(21)

The myocardium has a better opportunity for recovery when provided afterload reduction combined with augmented diastolic pressure.(16, 22) In addition, afterload reduction lowers the resistance to forward flow that enhances ventricular emptying, and therefore, increases cardiac output. Reductions in EDV further reduce myocardial oxygen demand by lowering ventricular wall tension. The resulting improvements in myocardial function allow further increases in cardiac output and end-organ perfusion. Thus, the IABP can reverse the ongoing deterioration that characterizes medically refractory cardiogenic shock.(23)

For the past 25 years, the largest subpopulation of IABP recipients has been those who undergo cardiac surgery and either cannot separate from cardiopulmonary bypass or experience cardiac failure during the early postoperative period. In the United States, postoperative IABP support is used in 2 to 12% of adult cardiac operations,(1, 14, 24–27) which accounts for 30 to 50% of all IABP applications.(28)

The majority of patients who receive post-cardiotomy IABP support can be weaned with subsequent 30-day and 2-year survival ranging from 52 to 65% and 42 to 56%, respectively (see Table 5C.3). Long-term survival differs little from patients with similar LV function who do not require IABP support,(25, 29) which corroborates clinical reviews that identify ventricular function as the most influential prognostic factor for post-cardiotomy patients.(30–32) Ventricular function, and therefore, patient outcome can be jeopardized when IABP therapy is not instituted expeditiously.(33–35) Some investigators have shown that "delaying" IABP therapy can increase mortality; "delay," however, requires further definition.(12,25,33,35,36) Timing becomes more dubious when IABP therapy manifests marginal results, and other mechanical circulatory support devices are considered. Therefore, predictors that would indicate the need for IABP therapy early on would be expected to have a positive impact on patient outcome.

Predicting the need for IABP support preoperatively has proved difficult if not impossible. Univariate, preoperative factors (ie, LV function, CHF, emergent operation) can estimate the likelihood for poor outcome following cardiac surgery.(37–43) However, the definitive need for post-cardiotomy IABP support can only be objectively determined when weaning from CPB. Most commonly, post-cardiotomy low-output syndromes result from pre-existing myocardial dysfunction, inadequate intraoperative myocardial protection, or perioperative myocardial infarction. Technical errors and prolonged cardiopulmonary bypass times can also be important contributing factors. In any case, hemodynamic criteria remain the only aid in identifying patients who need IABP support following cardiac surgery (see Table 5C.2). The initial criteria established nearly two decades ago (34) differ little from those used today. These standards can be easily confounded by a broadening array of pharmacologic regimens as well as the time intervals and techniques used to assess such therapy. And although the algorithm outlined earlier is used as a general guide by the cardiac team at Duke University Medical Center, universal protocols that outline a decisive approach to this critical decision process do not yet exist. This may, in part, explain that, although most patients receiving IABP for post-cardiotomy support experience successful reversal of their hemodynamic deterioration, mortality rates (approaching 50%) have changed little over more than a decade (1, 14, 24, 28, 44, 45) (see Table 5C.3). Clearly, the elucidation of objective criteria for the early identification of patients requiring post-cardiotomy IABP support would appear to have a positive impact on improving outcome in these challenging patients.

Review of the Duke experience substantiates these conclusions and raises other related questions regarding patients who require preoperative IABP support. During the 5-year period from January 1990 to December 1994, 6465 adult open heart procedures were performed at Duke University Medical Center. Of these cases, 523 (8.1%) received post-cardiotomy IABP support. However, only 194 (37%) experienced post-bypass hemodynamic instability as their indication for such therapy. The other 329 (63%) had the device continued empirically as an extension of its preoperative use. Not surprisingly, the 30-day mortality for patients receiving the IABP for post-bypass hemodynamic instability was relatively poor (31%). Furthermore, this mortality rate was relatively stable over the 5-year period with a range of 38% (high, 1990) to 25% (low, 1991). The mean 2-year survival in this group of patients was 42%, which is similar to results from other institutions (see Table 5C.3). In contrast, those patients who had a preoperative indication for IABP support experienced an average 30-day mortality of only 9.8%. Unfortunately, the 2-year survival data in these patients has not yet been analyzed. However, the 30-day mortality rate in patients with a preoperative indication for IABP support has trended downward, ranging from 17% (high, 1991) to 4% (low, 1994).

Careful examination of the Duke experience further highlights some other important trends regarding post-cardiotomy IABP utilization. Most notably, except for those patients with preoperative indications, the outcome for patients requiring post-pericardiotomy IABP support has remained relatively poor. Potential for improving these results may be found in either earlier IABP implementation through appropriately identified selection criteria and/or more aggressive use of ventricular assist devices (VADs). Undesirably, the selection criteria for VAD utilization in this setting is all the more ambiguous. Other equally important areas of controversy that have been noted in other series (14) relate to the preoperative utilization of IABP support. Of note, patients who receive preoperative IABP support represent the largest subgroup of postoperative IABP recipients at Duke. This subgroup not only enjoys a relatively favorable prognosis, but has demonstrated further improvements in outcome over the past 5 years. Therefore, one might question whether postoperative IABP support should be routinely implemented in these patients. In most cases where preoperative IABP support is used, the decision for post-cardiotomy support is, quite simply, empiric.

Preoperative Utilization of the IABP

Clearly, there are a number of settings in which the use of an IABP is indicated before urgent cardiac surgery. Probably the best examples are those patients who suffer acute myocardial infarction (MI) who meet hemodynamic criteria for cardiogenic shock. These patients experience a mortality of 100% when there is no improvement with medical therapy.(46) When the IABP first became clinically available, it was used most commonly for treating patients who experienced medically refractory shock secondary to MI.(47) In more than 75% of such cases, IABP support resulted in significant hemodynamic improvement.(48, 49) However, even today, survival for this group of patients remains consistently low unless interventions can be made to correct underlying pathology.(33, 50, 51) When IABP therapy leads to revascularization or repair of other underlying pathology, prognosis can be significantly improved.(28, 52) Therefore, the role of the IABP has significantly changed; today's approach is to use the IABP as an adjunct for other interventions. Approximately two thirds of patients who receive IABP therapy in this manner are found to have operable coronary anatomy. Thrombolysis and/or coronary angioplasty can acutely re-establish perfusion in a number of such cases and the decision for surgery can be made later. In other situations, the IABP provides a period of hemodynamic stabilization before emergent surgical revascularization. Survival following these strategies has been significantly improved in patients amenable to definitive therapy (14, 53, 54) compared with the high mortality in those with uncorrectable disease.

Other settings where the preoperative use of an IABP is indicated relate to the mechanical complications of acute myocardial infarction. Treatment options are relatively limited when support is required for an acutely ruptured ventricular septum or papillary muscle. Ischemic ventricular septal defect (VSD) or mitral valve regurgitation (MVR) demand early surgical intervention to avoid an otherwise exceedingly high mortality. Both MVR and VSD result from tissue necrosis,(14,53,54) which can complicate myocardial infarction in the intervening days or weeks after the event. The IABP can provide emergent, preoperative support when these complications occur,(55) whereas pharmacologic agents may be counterproductive. In the case of VSD, vasoconstrictors will further accentuate left-to-right shunting while afterload-reducing agents can further jeopardize coronary perfusion. The IABP is an ideal therapy because it decreases left-to-right shunting by lowering peak systolic pressures while augmenting diastolic pressures which, in turn, enhance myocardial perfusion.(56) In this manner, the IABP provides a critical period of hemodynamic stabilization that prepares the patient for surgery while minimizing risks of further cardiac or other end-organ damage. The mortality rates for VSD following acute MI has thereby been reduced from > 80% with no surgical intervention (57,58) to approximately 25% with successful VSD repair.(59,60) Finally, successful treatment of MVR following acute myocardial infarction has also been improved with use of IABP. This catastrophic event responds poorly to medical therapy. Inotropic agents that are used to restore contractility cause increases in afterload and myocardial oxygen consumption, which can exacerbate both mitral insufficiency and cardiac ischemia. As in the therapy of VSD, the IABP can reduce the mechanical impairment of MVR by reducing afterload while augmenting coronary blood flow through elevations in diastolic perfusion pressure.(61) Unfortunately, the surgical mortality for the treatment of this condition is nearly 50%, which is most likely related to the extent of underlying cardiac dysfunction.(62–65) While discouraging, these results represent a significant improvement compared with the > 90% overall mortality without surgical therapy.(66–70) There is some evidence that mitral repair as opposed to replacement may lead to better results in the treatment of MVR.(71) Irrespective of the choice of operative repair, the IABP is a valuable adjunct for the initial management of ischemic MVR or VSD.

Unlike the aforementioned indications, the increasing preoperative utilization of IABP support for myocardial ischemia refractory to medical therapy remains a somewhat controversial topic. In particular, the preoperative treatment of medically refractory ("unstable") angina using IABP support deserves some scrutiny. In general, unstable angina before surgical revascularization is associated with a poor prognosis.(72–75) This condition can occur in two groups of patients. One group has no evidence of myocardial infarction, termed preinfarction unstable angina, and the other is in convalescence from infarction, termed post-infarction unstable angina. IABP before revascularization may benefit patients in either group.(76–80) However, not all reports support this view,(81, 82) and only randomized clinical trials can definitively determine if such therapy favorably alters outcome. At present, preoperative IABP support has only been proved to benefit those patients whose condition before revascularization is complicated by hemodynamic instability.

While the preoperative use of IABP support of unstable angina may lend itself to further scrutiny, a much broader issue relates to the generally empiric use of post-cardiotomy IABP support in all patients who receive the IABP preoperatively. One might argue that all patients should undergo similar postoperative hemodynamic evaluations to ascertain the need for IABP support. Not unlike other previously outlined factors (see Table 5C.1), the need for IABP support in the preoperative setting might warrant a lower threshold for postoperative IABP use. However, empiric IABP use in all these cases may subject a significant number of patients to unnecessary risks without a clear benefit.

Conclusions

Although the IABP remains an invaluable adjunct for treating patients suffering from post-cardiotomy pump failure, its utility may be significantly enhanced by better defining selection criteria and indications. These goals would facilitate earlier implementation of IABP support when appropriate and, equally important, minimize the potential for unnecessary utilization. Only clinical trials can objectively determine the optimal therapeutic regimens before IABP insertion and whether or not preoperative IABP support should represent an indication for postoperative utilization. Until then, one risks subjecting patients to excessive doses of inotropic agents or unnecessary IABP support, both of which are attended by significant morbidity. Related issues that require equal attention revolve around the use of other mechanical circulatory support devices.(83) Because the IABP is generally considered a prerequisite to VADs, these matters become more complex and controversial when one attempts to discern the adequacy of IABP support vs the need for VAD therapy. When IABP support is insufficient, VADs have clearly proven effective but are associated with relatively high morbidity and mortality. Therefore, optimizing the complementary potential between IABP and VAD support is far more ambiguous. Resolution of these complex issues would most certainly lead to better patient outcome and cost effectiveness in the challenging treatment of post-cardiotomy pump failure.

REFERENCES

1. Pennington DG, Farrar DJ, Loisance D, Pae WEJ, Emery RW. Patient selection. Ann Thorac Surg 1993;55:206–212.
2. Haylor GDS, Hickey S, Bell G, Pei JM. Membrane oxygenators: Influence of design on performance. Perfusion 1995;9:173–190.
3. Burton AC. Physiology and biophysiology of the circulation. In: Burton, AC, ed. Chicago: Year Book Medical Publishers; 1972; pp 72, 207.
4. Kantrowitz A, McKinnon WMP. The experimental use of the diaphragm as an auxiliary myocardium. Surgical Forum 1959;9:265–267.
5. Harken DE. In: International College of Cardiology. Brussels, Belgium: 1958.
6. Clauss RH, Birtwell WC, Albertal G. Assisted Circulation. I. The arterial counterpulsator. J Thorac Cardiovasc Surg 1961;41:447.
7. Clauss RH, Misser P, Reed GE, Tice D. Assisted circulation by counterpulsation with intraaortic balloon. Methods and effects. In: Digest, 15th Annual Conference on Engineering in Medicine and Biology. Chicago: Northwestern University. 1962; p 44.
8. Moulopoulos SD, Topaz S, Kolff WJ. Diastolic balloon pumping (with carbon dioxide) in the aorta: Mechanical assistance to the failing circulation. Am Heart J 1962;63:669.
9. Sarnoff SJ, Braunwald E, Welch GHJ, Case RB, Stainsby WN, Macruz R. Hemodynamic determinants of oxygen consumption of the heart with special reference to the Tension-Time Index. Am J Physiol 1958;192:148–156.
10. Sheikh KH, Bengston JR, Rankin JS, deBruijn NP, Kisslo J. Intraoperative transesophageal doppler color flow imaging used to guide patient selection and operative treatment of ischemic mitral regurgitation. Circulation 1991;84:594–604.
11. Royster RL, et al. Combined inotropic effects of amrinone and epinephrine after cardiopulmonary bypass in humans. Anesth Analg 1993;77:662–672.
12. Pierce WS, Hershon JJ, Kormos RL, Dembitsky WP, Noon GP. Management of secondary organ dysfunction. Ann Thorac Surg 1993;55:222–226.
13. Loisance DY, et al. Pharmacological bridge to cardiac transplantation: Current limitations. Ann Thorac Surg 1993;55:310–313.
14. Naunheim KS, et al. Intraaortic balloon pumping in patients requiring cardiac operations. J Thorac Cardiovasc Surg 1992;104:1654–1661.

15. Hanloser PB, Gallow E, Schenk WG. Hemodynamics of counterpulsation. J Thorac Cardiovasc Surg 1966;51:366.

16. Bregman D. Mechanical support of the failing heart. In: Ravitch MM, ed. Current Problems in Surgery. Chicago: Year Book Medical Publishers; 1976.

17. Maroko PR, et al. Effects of intraaortic balloon counterpulsation on the severity of myocardial ischemic injury following acute coronary occlusion. Counterpulsation and myocardial injury. Circulation 1972;45:1150–1159.

18. Cox JL, Pass HI, Anderson RW, Wechsler AS, Oldham HN, Sabiston DC. Augmentation of coronary collateral blood flow in acute myocardial infarction. Surgical Forum 1975;26:238–240.

19. Buckley MJ, et al. Hemodynamic evaluation of intraaortic balloon pumping in man. Circulation 1970;41(suppl 5):II130-136.

20. Rose EA, Marrin CA, Bregman D, Spotnitz HM. Left ventricular mechanics of counterpulsation and left heart bypass, individually and in combination. J Thorac Cardiovasc Surg 1979;77:127–137.

21. Anstadt MP. Clinical experience using the IABP at Duke University Medical Center: A five year experience. Unpublished; 1995.

22. Corday E, et al. Physiologic principles in the application of circulatory assist for the failing heart. Intraaortic balloon circulatory assist and venoarterial phased partial bypass. Am J Cardiol 1970;26:595–602.

23. Scheidt S, et al. Intra-aortic balloon counterpulsation in cardiogenic shock. Report of a co-operative clinical trial. N Engl J Med 1973;288:979–984.

24. DiLello F, Mullen DC, Flemma RJ, Anderson AJ, Kleinman LH, Werner PH. Results of intraaortic balloon pumping after cardiac surgery: Experience with the Percor balloon catheter. Ann Thorac Surg 1988;46:442–446.

25. Golding LAR, Loop FD, Peter M, Cosgrove DM, Taylor PC, Phillips DF. Late survival following use of intraaortic balloon pump in revascularization operations. Ann Thorac Surg 1980;30:48–51.

26. Creswell LL, et al. Intraaortic balloon counterpulsation: Patterns of usage and outcome in cardiac surgery patients. Ann Thorac Surg 1992;54:11–20.

27. Baldwin RT, et al. A model to predict survival at time of postcardiotomy intraaortic balloon pump insertion. Ann Thorac Surg 1993;55:908–913.

28. Bolooki H. Current status of circulatory support with an intra-aortic balloon pump. Cardiology Clin 1985;3:123–133.

29. Davies R, Laks H, Berger H. Follow-up radionuclide assessment of left ventricular function and perfusion in patients requiring intraaortic balloon pump to wean from cardiopulmonary bypass. Am J Cardiol 1980;45:488.

30. Force T, et al. Perioperative myocardial infarction after coronary artery bypass surgery. Clinical significance and approach to risk stratification. Circulation 1990;82:903–912.

31. Myers WO, et al. Improved survival of surgically treated patients with triple vessel coronary artery disease and severe angina pectoris. A report from the Coronary Artery Surgery Study (CASS) registry. J Thorac Cardiovasc Surg 1989;97:487–495.

32. Lytle BW, et al. Fifteen hundred coronary reoperations. Results and determinants of early and late survival. J Thorac Cardiovasc Surg 1987;93:847–859.

33. Bolooki H, et al. Clinical and hemodynamic criteria for use of the intra-aortic balloon pump in patients requiring cardiac surgery. J Thorac Cardiovasc Surg 1976;72:756–768.

34. Norman JC, et al. Prognostic indices for survival during postcardiotomy intraaortic balloon pumping. Methods of scoring and classification, with implications for left ventricular assist device utilization. J Thorac Cardiovasc Surg 1977;74:709–720.

35. Anstadt MP, et al. Intraoperative timing may provide criteria for use of postcardiotomy ventricular assist devices. ASAIO J 1992;38:M147–M150.

36. Parascandola SA, Pae WE, Davis PK, Miller CA, Pierce WS, Waldhausen JA. Determinants of survival in patients with ventricular assist devices. ASAIO Trans 1988;34:222–228.

37. Chaitman BR, Ryan TJ, Kronmal RA, Foster ED, Frommer PL, Killip T. Coronary Artery Surgery Study (CASS): Comparability of 10 year survival in randomized and randomizable patients. J Am Coll Cardiol 1990;16:1071–1078.

38. Edwards FH, et al. True emergency coronary artery bypass surgery. Ann Thorac Surg 1990;49:603–610.

39. Sergeant P, Wouters L, Dekeyser L, Flameng W, Suy R. Is the outcome of coronary artery bypass graft surgery predictable in patients with severe ventricular function impairment? J Cardiovasc Surg 1986;27:618–621.

40. Alder DS, et al. Long-term survival of more than 2,000 patients after coronary artery bypass grafting. Am J Cardiol 1986;58:195–202.

41. Freed PS, Wasfie T, Zado B, Kantrowitz A. Intraaortic balloon pumping for prolonged circulatory support. Am J Cardiol 1988;61:554–557.

42. Miller DC, et al. Discriminant analysis of the changing risks of coronary artery operations: 1971-1979. J Thorac Cardiovasc Surg 1983;85:197–213.

43. Brahos GJ, et al. Aortocoronary bypass following unsuccessful PTCA: Experience in 100 consecutive patients. Ann Thorac Surg 1985;40:7–10.

44. Gottlieb SO, et al. Identification of patients at high risk for complications of intraaortic balloon counterpulsation: A multivariate risk factor analysis. Am J Cardiol 1984;53:1135–1139.

45. Wasfie T, et al. Risks associated with intraaortic balloon pumping in patients with and without diabetes mellitus. Am J Cardiol 1988;61:558–562.

46. Scheidt S, Ascheim R, Killip T. Shock after acute myocardial infarction: A clinical and hemodynamic profile. Am J Cardiol 1970;26:556.

47. Weber KT, Janicki JS. Intraaortic balloon counterpulsation. Ann Thorac Surg 1974;17:602–636.

48. Dunkman WB, et al. Clinical and hemodynamic results of intraaortic balloon pumping and surgery for cardiogenic shock. Circulation 1972;46:465–477.

49. Levine FH, Austen WG. Intraaortic balloon assistance. In: Glenn WWL, ed. Thoracic and Cardiovascular Surgery. Norwalk, Conn: Appleton-Century-Crofts; 1983;p 1157.

50. Allen BS, et al. Studies on prolonged acute regional ischemia IV. Myocardial infarction with left ventricular power failure: A medical surgical emergency requiring urgent revascularization with maximal protection of remote muscle. J Thorac Cardiovasc Surg 1989;98:691–703.

51. Bolooki H. Emergency cardiac procedures in patients in cardiogenic shock due to complications of coronary artery disease. Circulation 1989; 79(suppl 1):137–148.

52. Pennington DG, Swartz MT, Codd JE, Merjavy JP, Kaiser GC. Intraaortic balloon pumping in cardiac surgical patients: A nine-year experience. Ann Thorac Surg 1983;36:125–131.

53. McEnany MT, Kay HR, Buckley MJ. Clinical experience with intraaortic balloon pump support in 728 patients. Circulation 1978;58(suppl I):1–24.

54. Pierri MK, et al. Exercise tolerance in late survivors of balloon pumping and surgery for cardiogenic shock. Circulation 1980;62(2:Pt 2):I138–I141.

55. Heitmiller R, Jacobs ML, Dagget WM. Surgical management of postinfarction ventricular septal rupture. Ann Thorac Surg 1986;41:683.

56. Gold HK, Leinbach RC, Sanders CA, Buckley MJ, Mundth ED, Austen WG. Intraaortic balloon pumping for ventricular septal defect or mitral regurgitation complicating acute myocardial infarction. Circulation 1973;47:1191–1196.

57. Sanders RJ, Kern WH, Blount SG. Perforation of the interventricular septum complicating myocardial infarction. Am Heart J 1956;51:736.

58. Oyamada A, Queen FB. Spontaneous rupture of the interventricular septum following acute myocardial infarction with some clinicopathologic observations on survival in five cases. In: Tripler Hospital Publication: First Pan-Pacific Pathology Congress. US Army Hospital, Honolulu, Hawaii; 1961.

59. Gaudiani VA, et al. Postinfarction ventricular septal defect: An argument for early operation. Surgery 1981;89:48–55.

60. Daggett WM, Buckley WJ, Akins CW. Improved results of surgical management of postinfarction ventricular septal rupture. Ann Surg 1982;196: 269–277.

61. Mueller H, Ayres SM, Giannelli SJ, Conklin EF, Mazzara JT, Grace WJ. Cardiac performance and metabolism in shock due to acute myocardial infarction in man: Response to catecholamines and mechanical cardiac assist. Trans NY Acad Sci 1972;34:309–333.

62. Tepe NA, Edmunds LHJ. Operation for acute postinfarction mitral insufficiency and cardiogenic shock. J Thorac Cardiovasc Surg 1985;89:525.

63. Radford MJ, Johnson RA, Buckley MJ, Daggett WM, Leinbach RC, Gold HK. Survival following mitral valve replacement for mitral regurgitation due to coronary artery disease. Circulation 1979;60(2:Pt 2):39–47.

64. Magovern JA, Pennock JL, Campbell DB, Pierce WS, Waldhausen JA. Risks of mitral valve replacement and mitral valve replacement with coronary artery bypass. Ann Thorac Surg 1985;39:346–352.

65. DiSesa VJ, Cohn LH, Collins JJ Jr, Koster JK Jr, VanDevanter S. Determinants of operative survival following combined mitral valve replacement and coronary revascularization. Ann Thorac Surg 1982;34:482–489.

66. Sanders RJ, Neubuerger KT, Ravin A. Rupture of papillary muscles. Occurrence of rupture of the posterior muscle and posterior myocardial infarction. Dis Chest 1957;31:316.

67. Wei JY, Hutchins GM, Bulkley BM. Papillary muscle rupture and fatal acute myocardial infarction. Ann Intern Med 1979;90:149.

68. DePasquale NP, Burch GE. Papillary muscle dysfunction in coronary (ischemic) heart disease. Annu Rev Med 1971;22:327.

69. DeBusk RF, Harrison DC. The clinical spectrum of papillary-muscle disease. N Engl J Med 1969;281:1458.

70. Morrow AG, Cohen LS, Roberts WC, Braunwald NS, Braunwald E. Severe mitral regurgitation following acute myocardial infarction and ruptured papillary muscle. Hemodynamic findings and results of operative treatment in four patients. Circulation 1968;37(suppl 4):II124–132.

71. Connolly MW, et al. Surgical results for mitral regurgitation from coronary artery disease. J Thorac Cardiovasc Surg 1986;91:379–388.
72. Fulton M, et al. Natural history of unstable angina. Lancet I 1972:860–865.
73. Gazes PC, Mobley EMJ, Faris HM Jr, Duncan RC, Humphries GB. Preinfarctional (unstable) angina–a prospective study–ten year follow-up. Prognostic significance of electrocardiographic changes. Circulation 1973;48:331–337.
74. Fischl SJ, Herman MJ, Gorlin R: The intermediate coronary syndrome. Clinical, angiographic and therapeutic aspects. N Engl J Med 288:1193, 1973.
75. Schuster EH, Bulkley BH. Early postinfarction angina. N Engl J Med 1981;305:1101.
76. Harris PL, Woollard K, Bartoli A, Makey AR. The management of impending myocardial infarction using coronary bypass grafting and an intraaortic balloon pump. J Cardiovasc Surg 1980;21:405–408.
77. Levine FH, Gold HK, Leinbach RC. Management of acute myocardial ischemia with intraaortic balloon pumping and surgery. Circulation 1978;58(suppl I):1–69.
78. Gold HK, Leinbach RC, Buckley MJ, Mundth ED, Daggett WM, Austen WG. Refractory angina pectoris: Follow-up after intraaortic balloon pumping and surgery. Circulation 1976;54(suppl III):III41–III46.
79. Bardet J, Rigaud M, Kahn JC, Huret JF, Gandjbakhch I, Bourdarias JP. Treatment of post-myocardial infarction angina by intra-aortic balloon pumping and emergency revascularization. J Thorac Cardiovasc Surg 1977;74:299–306.
80. Creswell LL, Moulton MJ, Cox JL, Rosenbloom M. Revascularization after acute myocardial infarction. Ann Thorac Surg 1995;60:19–26.
81. Brundage BH, Ullyot DJ, Winokur S, Chatterjee K, Ports TA, Turley K. The role of aortic balloon pumping in postinfarction angina. A different perspective. Circulation 1980;62:1119–1123.
82. Williams DB, Ivey TD, Bailey WW, Irey SJ, Rideout JT, Stewart D. Postinfarction angina: Results of early revascularization. J Am Coll Cardiol 1983;2:859–864.
83. Anstadt MP, Lowe JE. The coronary circulation: Surgical management of coronary artery disease: Assisted circulation. In: Spencer S, ed. Surgery of the Chest. Philadelphia: WB Saunders; 1995, pp 1995–2016.

6

Complications of Intra-aortic Balloon Pump Therapy

Andrea P. Baldyga, M.D.

Introduction

The intra-aortic balloon pump (IABP) has proved to be an invaluable aid to the operative and nonoperative management of cardiovascular disorders since its clinical introduction in 1968. Shortly after the balloon pump's introduction, however, its own impact in contributing to morbidity and mortality was realized. Over the succeeding years several changes have been implemented in the insertion technique and design of the device in order to make it more usable by a more diverse group of medical practitioners, as well as to attempt to decrease the potential for complications. The most notable of these changes was the introduction of the percutaneous IABP in 1979. Despite its ease of insertion, it too proved to have many problems associated with its use. Since then, the wire-guided percutaneous balloon catheter has been developed, as well as devices with smaller diameter catheters as further approaches to decrease complications. While the initial IABP catheters were single-lumen 14 French (Fr) and required surgical insertion, advances in technology today have provided the percutaneous 9.5 Fr double-lumen, and 8.5 Fr single-lumen catheters, which are the most commonly used versions today. Although the incidence of some complications has changed, the use of the device still requires the practitioner to be aware of the possible problems, and to assess the risk-benefit ratio for each patient in whom the intra-aortic balloon pump is used.

The most common complications encountered throughout the balloon pump's clinical history have been vascular, with vascular occlusion at the site of entry due to arterial injury or thrombosis around the catheter the most prevalent. Other major complications include the distal mechanical catastrophes of aortic dissection and vascular perforation. Infection, particularly at the site of insertion of the IABP, can also be a source of morbidity. These complications, as well as many that are less frequent, along with their diagnosis, prevention, and management, will be discussed in this chapter. Hopefully, this will give the clinician the necessary information based on the experience of others to avoid some complications or to deal with them in a more effective manner.

Vascular Complications

In order to look at the major complications associated with IABP use most rationally, it is useful to break down the reported clinical experience into roughly three time periods related to the changes that have been made in balloon pump design and technology. The first era is from the introduction in 1968 of the first IABP for clinical use until the development of the percutaneous catheter in 1979. The period of the percutaneous catheter's use was fairly brief, because shortly thereafter a percutaneous wire-guided catheter was developed that is the most commonly used catheter today.

There is difficulty in analyzing the incidence of complications due to varying definitions of complications by different authors. Some series include the extraction of asymptomatic clot at routine thrombectomy during removal of the IABP as a vascular complication, whereas others do not. Because the reported incidence of "bland" thrombus at balloon removal is as high as 64%,(1) this can obviously cause great difficulty in data analysis. Some authors report complications based on the total number of insertions as opposed to survivors, which because of the overall mortality due to the underlying cardiovascular disease can be significant. The exclusion of patients in whom balloon insertion is unsuccessful also affects the results as higher incidence of complications has been reported in patients who have attempted but unsuccessful insertions.(2) Nonetheless, some basic trends regarding the complications of the procedure can be derived.

Early Experience

The earliest IABPs were 12 or 14 Fr catheters that required formal surgical insertion through a vascular graft sutured to a common femoral arteriotomy. When the balloon pump was removed, the graft could either be amputated close to the arteriotomy and oversewn, or totally removed with primary repair of the artery to avoid the potential complications of prosthetic material in a contaminated wound. At the time of removal, may surgeons routinely performed Fogarty thrombectomy proximally and distally to remove any possibility for later thrombosis and embolus.

Although complications associated with the IABP were initially reported to be negligible,(3) further experience with the device began to show an increasing occurrence of several different problems. The overall incidence of complications ranged from 17 to 36% in several series, with the majority reporting an approximately 25% complication rate. Inability to insert the balloon through the usual femoral approach generally occurred between 5 and 10% of the time (range, 2.4 to 21%).(2, 4–6) In some cases, other approaches, such as ascending aorta, iliac, or subclavian access achieved successful placement. The use of alternate sites for IABP insertion will be discussed in detail later in the chapter. Catastrophic arterial perforation occurred in less than 1% of patients, most of whom died secondary to the complication.(2, 5, 7, 8) Lethal arterial dissection also occurred in approximately 1% of insertions.(5–9) In patients who were able to communicate the most common symptom of dissection was back pain; limb ischemia was also noted. Interestingly, although the occurrence of many dissections was recognized as a disastrous event, many cases were able to be treated simply by IABP removal with a subsequent benign course (2, 5, 10). Recognition occurred only in retrospect at the time of angiography, cardiac surgery, balloon pump removal, or at autopsy. Isner et al, in a study of 45 IABP patients who underwent necropsy, found a 36% incidence of complications, only 20% of which had been suspected antemortem.(11) The most common complication found was arterial dissection accounting for 20% of the entire series. In none of these instances was the dissection suspected or diagnosed before death. There was no difficulty at all reported with insertion in half of these cases, and in 20% of the dissection patients, there was hemodynamic improvement with good wave form display and balloon function despite the location of the balloon entirely in the false lumen. There is also a report of aortic dissection contiguous to the site of the inflating balloon that occurred without evidence of any intimal injury, presumably due to shear force on the aorta.(12) Therefore, the possibility of dissection must always be considered as a cause of unexplained hemodynamic instability in patients during or after IABP therapy, even in whom there has been no evidence of difficulty at insertion or during pumping.

The majority of complications were related to vascular ischemia, with most reports finding an incidence of between 8 to 15% (range, 2.4–36%). (1, 2, 4–10) Between a third and a half of these patients required operative repair of the ischemia, most needing only thrombectomy and/or local repair for intimal flap at the site of insertion, but some patients required more extensive repair that was not always successful in obviating the ischemic damage, which necessitated fasciotomy and amputation in 1 to 2%. Early or late hemorrhage from the groin site occurred in less than 3% of patients. Late pseudoaneurysm development also occurred, but was quite rare. Lymphocele or prolonged lymph drainage was a source of morbidity in some patients, and contributed to some episodes of late sepsis.(8) Overall IABP associated mortality was 1% in most series, although Pace reported mortality of 4.8% in a series of 104 patients.(7) The majority of the deaths were related to the catastrophic complications previously mentioned; in addition, patients died of gangrenous bowel and spinal ischemia.(7, 9)

Different authors found various factors to be associated with complications. Lefemine et al reported a 50% incidence of complications, primarily ischemia, in patients in cardiogenic shock.(4) Pace noted that 47% of complications occurred in patients with pre-existing peripheral vascular disease (PVD), and that the incidence of these complications was related to the duration of IABP support.(7) On the other hand, Perler and co-workers found that 95% of the patients who sustained a vascular complication in his series of nearly 800 patients denied any pre-insertion history of symptoms of vascular disease and that 78% of these patients had normal pulses before insertion, despite the frequent finding of significant disease at the time of insertion.(8) Therefore, although a history of peripheral vascular disease may be a risk factor for the development of vascular problems, the absence of such a history does not obviate the risk of complications. McEnany et al saw increased vascular and infectious problems with longer length of balloon therapy, whereas Macoviak et al reported only increased infections with longer support.(5, 9) Beckman found complications to be associated with difficult insertion, and McCabe found a higher incidence of complications in patients who had IABP insertion attempted unsuccessfully than in patients who had experienced successful insertion.(2, 10)

Advent of the Percutaneous IABP

In an attempt to decrease the incidence of these complications as well as to increase the speed and efficiency with which the IABP could be inserted, the first percutaneous IABP was released for clinical use in 1979. Insertion of an introducer sheath was performed by the percutaneous Seldinger technique, with the 12 Fr balloon catheter then inserted via the sheath into the artery. The initial reports of the use of this technique found few complications, and there was a marked decrease in the amount of time needed for IABP assistance to be instituted.(13–15) The percutaneous device could be inserted in less than 5 minutes and did not require the services of a vascular surgeon or a formal arterial procedure. As the technique was more widely performed, however, complications were reported, and comparisons were made of the results and complications of the surgical and percutaneous balloon catheters.(16–21) Although the ease with which the catheter could be inserted was an advantage in emergency settings, there was not a significant difference in the ability to insert the balloon with the percutaneous rather than the surgical technique,

Table 6.1

Comparison of Surgical vs Percutaneous (Nonm-Wire Guided)
IABP Insertion[a]

IABP Complications	Surgical (n =201) (%)	Percutaneous (n = 161) (%)
Aortoiliac rupture	0.5	2.5
Aortoiliac dissection	0.5	1.2
Ischemia	4.8	9.3
Wound infection	3.0	1.2

[a]*Reprinted with permission from Pennington DG et al. Intra-aortic balloon pumping in cardiac surgical patients: A nine year experience. Ann Thorac Surg 1983;36:125–131.*

successful insertion being accomplished in between 90 and 95% of all patients.(16, 19, 22) The rate of most major complications for the percutaneous technique was almost double that of surgical insertion in most studies (Table 6.1). Dissection occurred in 2% of percutaneous patients as compared with 1% or less of surgical patients. (16–18) The rate of arterial perforation was also more than doubled, occurring in greater than 2% of patients undergoing the percutaneous technique, and in 0.5% or less of surgical patients.(16–18) Significant ischemia (most cases requiring surgical intervention) occurred in 5 to 30% of percutaneous patients, and in 1 to 12% of surgical patients.(16–19, 21, 23, 24) Asymptomatic loss of pulses, which was remedied merely by removal of the IABP, occurred in approximately the same number of patients, but was generally considered a minor complication.(19) The requirement for amputation was approximately 1%. Although the majority of vascular complications occurred during pumping, there was noted to be an increased incidence of complications at the time of removal, or later. This was thought to be due to the effect of the "bland" thrombus seen at removal in earlier reports. Goldman et al, confirming Alpert's earlier report, found asymptomatic thrombus in 20% of patients at the time of surgical removal.(1, 16) Reasons for increased vascular complications with the percutaneous technique include the potential for unwitting local intimal dissection, particularly in the diseased artery, which can be propagated proximally with further advancement of the balloon catheter. Diseased or tortuous iliac arteries can cause the rather stiff balloon catheter to dissect or freely perforate the artery at that level as well. The inability to accurately cannulate the common femoral artery can cause thrombosis of the smaller superficial femoral artery, and it is not possible to remove the thrombus that not infrequently occurs at the site of cannulation, particularly in a smaller artery, via the percutaneous technique.

Although vascular problems were increased, the problem of infection was significantly decreased by avoiding the necessity for femoral cutdown. The incidence of wound infections was negligible in most series with the percutaneous technique (16, 17, 19) but bleeding and hematoma most often related to removal was higher than that of surgical balloons (2 vs 1%).(16) Although the overall IABP-related mortality remained low at less than 2% in most series, with many authors not reporting any mortality in their series, there were more deaths secondary to the major complications of perforation and dissection, which occurred with higher frequency in percutaneous patients.(17, 18)

With more experience in the use and complications of the percutaneous IABP, several authors attempted to find correlations and predictors of balloon pump morbidity and mortality, some of which corresponded with the findings from the earlier surgical experience. Goldman and co-workers, commenting on a series of 299 patients, found an increased incidence of complications in patients with peripheral vascular disease (PVD) insertions that were difficult or performed while the patient was in cardiogenic shock, or required prolonged IABP support.(16) Gottlieb et al, who surveyed the results in 101 surgical and 105 percutaneous patients, found female gender, peripheral vascular disease, and percutaneous technique to be significant by multivariate analysis. There was a threefold risk of vascular problems in patients with PVD compared with those without.(19) For women without PVD, there was a fourfold increase in risk, presumably secondary to the smaller size of women's arteries, which are more easily obstructed by the introducer sheath and balloon catheter itself; this increase was canceled out in the presence of pre-existing vascular disease. Percutaneous insertion increased the risk of vascular complications in both genders twofold. Shahian and co-workers, writing in 1983, was similarly struck by the difference in vascular complication rates in men and women.(18) Seventy-one percent of women who had catheters inserted percutaneously incurred vascular complications vs 10% in men, whereas there was a lack of gender difference in complications in surgically inserted balloons. He advised that the surgical technique should always be used in women to decrease the risk of complications, although the percutaneous technique was safer in men. Kantrowitz et al, looking at his entire experience of 733 patients comprising primarily surgical, but also including percutaneous insertions, confirmed the increased risk of IABP in female patients (32 vs 18% complications, F:M), but also noted the deleterious effect of diabetes and hypertension, both of which have a high level of correlation with PVD, but vascular disease *per se* was not a predictor of complication in this large series.(22) He also found no relation of problems to the presence of shock at insertion, or the duration of balloon pumping. To specifically study the impact of diabetes on balloon-related morbidity, Wasfie and co-workers studied a series of 132 diabetic patients who had undergone IABP placement and compared them with a group of nondiabetics.(25) Successful insertion was obtained in 95% of both groups. The incidence of vascular complications was highest in insulin-dependent diabetes mellitus (IDDM) vs non–insulin-dependent diabetes mellitus (NIDDM) and nondiabetic patients (34 vs 18% vs 14%, respectively). Wound infections were similarly increased, with 23% of IDDM patients, 4% of NIDDM and 4% of nondiabetics suffering this complication. Despite these complications, however, the hospital survival of diabetics was the same as that of non-diabetics, so that continued use of this modality is warranted in the diabetic patient population.

Because of the association of complications at the time of insertion and removal of the balloon catheter, many authors attempted to find safer techniques. Vignola et al reported on the use of a longer introducer sheath, which when inserted properly by the Seldinger technique appeared to more safely negotiate the often tortuous and diseased distal iliac and femoral arteries.(26) He also stressed meticulous attention to the maintenance of pressure to the insertion site in the groin after removal using a compression clamp that appeared to be more reliable than manual pressure. In his series of 54 patients, 10.2% developed femoral thrombosis, 80% of whom required thrombectomy. There were no occurrences of dissection, pseudoaneurysm or groin hematomas. The other approach that has been taken to the problem of balloon removal has been surgical exploration and removal of even percutaneously placed balloons as reported by Cutler et al.(27) This allows for Fogarty thrombectomy, and thus removal of the clot, which could lead to vascular occlusion at the time of, or following, balloon removal, as well as the securing of hemostasis. In his series, this technique eliminated vascular complications in the surgically explored group, whereas the percutaneously removed group sustained 10.5% hemorrhagic, and 21% thrombotic complications.

Recent Experience with the Percutaneous Wire-Guided IABP

Most recently, a double-lumen intra-aortic balloon pump has been developed that allows for percutaneous insertion of the balloon catheter itself over a wire positioned in the descending aorta. The aim of this technology was to increase the rate of successful cannulation and to aid in the prevention of the complications of dissection and perforation due to the tortuosity and disease in the arterial tree. Successful insertion has been reported in between 90 and 100% of insertions.(28, 29) Unfortunately, the incidence of vascular complications has not improved significantly. The comment is made in several papers that making negotiation of tortuous and diseased arteries easier may, in fact, predispose for an increased incidence of later ischemia, because cannulation can now be achieved in arteries that would earlier have been inaccessible for balloon pump placement. The incidence of ischemia ranges between 9 and 43%, with the need for surgical correction in one third to one half of these cases.(29–32) Amputation is still required for irreversible limb ischemia in 0.5 to 1.5% of patients.(31, 32) Dissection and perforation appear to have decreased, with only two recent studies (33, 34) reporting 1.3 to 1.4% dissection, and 0.5 to 0.7% perforation. Several other recent articles have not noted any occurrences of these catastrophic complications. (29, 31, 32) Pseudoaneurysm formation has decreased to 1% or less (31, 35) and bleeding or hematoma at the groin site continues to occur in less than 3% of patients following IABP removal. (31, 32, 34)

With the development of percutaneous balloons, the use of graft material for insertion of the catheter for open insertion through the femoral artery is not generally required. Whether wire-guided or not, the balloon can easily be inserted through a purse string suture, with or without the introducer sheath, into the arterial system. Open removal is usually obligated because of the risk of hemorrhage at removal. An alternative technique that avoids the use of the potentially obstructing sheath, as well as the risks of prosthetic material in the wound, is the use of a short segment of saphenous vein left over from coronary bypass, or harvested at the time of balloon insertion. At the time of removal, the vein is simply ligated flush to the artery. Percutaneous IABPs have been inserted without a sheath (36, 37) and recently, balloon catheters specifically designed for sheathless percutaneous insertion have been developed in an attempt to make the catheter profile as low as possible, which may be of importance, particularly in small arteries. Initial reports of both techniques appear promising with Tatar reporting a vascular complication rate of only 8.8% in patients having balloon pump insertion without a sheath compared with 25.9% of patients with conventional insertion.(37) Approximately half of patients in each group required operative intervention. An initial trial of this new design of IABP for percutaneous insertion reported a 10% incidence of ischemia.(38)

Because the intra-aortic balloon pump has now been available for clinical use for 25 years, a wide breadth of experience in its use has developed. Several recent studies have looked at the longitudinal experience with balloon pumping in an attempt to find better predictors of its utility as well as risk. Naunheim et al and Barnett et al have reported on the most recent 7-year experience at St. Louis University, comprising a group of 580 patients who had undergone cardiac surgery.(39, 40) The insertion techniques included 65% percutaneous, and 35% by an open technique, with or without a vascular graft. The overall complication rate was 12.4%, of which 49% required operative intervention (5.8% of the total group). Ischemia occurred in 11.9%, aortic perforation in 0.5%, with an IABP-related death rate of 0.5% (all of the patients who had suffered perforation). Multivariate analysis disclosed six independent predictors of mortality: preoperative New York Heart Association (NYHA) class, transthoracic bal-

Table 6.2

Clinical Experience at St. Louis University Hospital, 1972 to 1990[a]		
	1972–1981 (n = 378) (%)	1982–1990 (n = 580) (%)
IABP complications		
Minor	5.8	9.8
Major	5.8	2.5
IABP-related mortality	2.1	0.5
Hospital mortality	46.6	44

[a]Reprinted with permission from Naunheim, KS, et al. Intra-aortic balloon pumping in patients requiring cardiac operations. Risk analysis and long-term follow-up. J Thorac Cardiovasc Surg 1992;104:1654–1661.

loon insertion, preoperative administration of nitroglycerin (improved mortality), age, female gender, preoperative balloon insertion (improved mortality compared to intraoperative or postoperative insertion). The presence of these variables, however, were only weak predictors of mortality. The occurrence of balloon-related complications was not predictive of death. In comparing this group of patients to their previous 9-year experience (1972–1981) (Table 6.2), although the total number of complications was the same (11.6 vs 12.4%), the number of major vascular complications had decreased (2.5 vs 5.8%), as had the IABP-related death rate (0.5 vs 2.1%) (see Table 6.2) Despite this improvement, the overall hospital mortality rate was unchanged (44 vs 46.6%). Thus improvement in technique, experience, and balloon pump technology have contributed to a decrease in balloon-related effects on mortality, but the underlying disease process responsible for the need for the IABP remains the same.

Makhoul et al surveyed the 14-year experience in 436 patients who underwent IABP placement at Duke University.(41) The incidence of vascular complications was 10.6%; 90% of patients with these complications required operative intervention. (One suspects that these researchers used a more rigorous definition of ischemia to account for this high percentage of patients who required operation than that in most other series, which reported a 30 to 50% necessity for surgery.) Dissection occurred in 0.46%, and bleeding requiring operative repair in 0.69%. The only predictor of vascular complications was the absence of pedal pulses on admission. Female gender was not a predictor of morbidity.

A recent longitudinal study by Alle found female gender and pre-existing peripheral vascular disease to be significant risk factors for the development of their 33% incidence of vascular complications during a 10-year period.(42) Insertion site, the technique or difficulty of insertion, age and duration of counterpulsation did not affect the incidence of vascular complications. Miller and co-workers, who reported on the most recent 3-year experience at Emory University, found an 18.3% incidence of vascular complications, 55% of whom required operation.(35) Risk factors for development of these complications included diminished or absent femoral pulses on initial examination, female gender, and obesity. The combination of peripheral vascular disease and percutaneous insertion increased the vascular morbidity twofold as compared with the cut-down technique. In contrast to most other studies, including that of Naunheim, these researchers found the mortality rate in the presence of vascular complications to be double that of patients without vascular complications (34 vs 17%). In a study specifically surveying the risk of IABP in relation to peripheral vascular disease, Kvilekval et al found an overall incidence of vascular complications of 12%, consistent with most series, but the incidence of vascular complications was 60% in patients with PVD, and 5% in those without.(33) He further divided the vascular patients into those with aneurysmal disease and occlusive disease. There was a 4.2% incidence of both embolic and occlusive complications for the entire group. Emboli were found to occur in 20% of patients with PVD as compared with 1.5% in the patients without PVD, and vascular occlusion in 25% of PVD patients in comparison to 0.8% of non-PVD patients. In the embolic group, all of the patients with PVD had aneurysmal disease, whereas in the occlusion group, all the PVD patients had atherosclerotic occlusive disease. Only one patient with a known preoperative ankle/brachial index of <1.0 did not have a complication. The associated mortality with emboli was 50%, whereas there were no associated deaths with occlusive complications. Technical complications ensued more frequently in the PVD group (15 vs 3%), but there was no associated mortality. Overall mortality was not statistically significant between those with vascular disease and those without (30% in PVD, 15% in non-PVD).

Insertion of IABP Through Pre-existing Vascular Grafts

The presence of a pre-existing aortofemoral vascular graft was initially considered a contraindication to placement of an IABP via the femoral approach, requiring ascending aortic, or other more unusual cannulation. Experience from vascular radiology has shown that it is possible to cannulate Dacron femoral grafts without significant morbidity.(43) The first report of the use of cannulation of aortofemoral graft for IABP insertion is from 1988 by Shahian and co-workers, who placed side-arm grafts, similar to the previous method of open cannulation, onto two recent graft (one 2 months, and one 6 days after vascular surgery).(44) Reports since then have confirmed the safety of this approach.(45, 46) LaMuraglia et al also used percutaneous cannulation of mature grafts, and reserved open techniques for recently placed grafts.(46) Three patients developed limb ischemia (16%), all of whom had percutaneous placement via a mature graft. Two of these patients required later thrombectomy, whereas one patient's condition resolved without operation. There were no infections, bleeding, or pseudoaneurysms. There was one death, possibly related to disruption of a fresh vascular anastomosis, but no autopsy was obtained to confirm the diagnosis. Thus, when necessary the IABP can be placed with reasonable safety in patients with Dacron femoral grafts.

Insertion Through the Ascending Aorta

The use of the ascending aorta as the site for IABP insertion was first reported by Gueldner and Lawrence in 1975.(47) The indication for its use was the inability to pass the balloon catheter through severely diseased distal arteries. Since then, many authors have reported use of this technique not only in cases of severe peripheral arterial disease, but, in some series, as the preferred method of intraoperative insertion.(48, 49) Another indication for the transthoracic technique is the presence of abdominal aortic aneurysm, and earlier in the IABP experience, in patients who had undergone previous aortofemoral grafts. An advantage of this approach is the quick and direct access to the aorta in the event of hemodynamic instability with the chest opened in the operating room. Obviously, insertion via the ascending aorta requires operative exposure, but removal techniques have been reported that use a vascular graft that can be tunneled through the chest wall and left in the subcutaneous tissues, which allows for later removal in the intensive care unit (ICU) with only a local exploration, obviating the need for reoperation.(50–54) (Fig. 6.1) This approach would have the advantage of decreasing the risk attendant with another operative procedure and anesthetic in already critically ill patients, as well as to potentially lower the incidence of mediastinitis and sternal wound problems. Other authors have used simple pursestring sutures to insert the IABP, much in the same fashion that operative aortic cannulation is secured.(47, 55, 56) (Fig. 6.2) A reported problem with the suture technique was inadequate fixation of an IABP leading to partial extrusion of the balloon from the aorta leading to hemorrhage during balloon diastole.(57)

Questions have been raised regarding the ultimate safety of this approach, particularly the concern for neurologic complications due to the necessity of passage of the balloon past the arch vessels at the time of insertion and removal in patients with known atherosclerotic disease. In attempt to prevent this complication, Bonchek et al recommended open removal of the balloon with snare occlusion of the head vessels as the catheter is being withdrawn.(55) Although this approach makes sense, there has been no reported widespread use of the technique. The reported incidence of all complications with this procedure have actually been surprisingly low. Pennington and Pelletier reported no complications in a

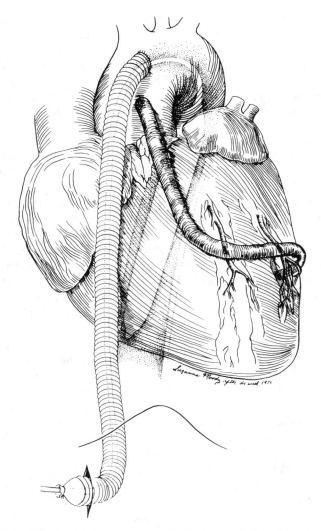

Figure 6.1. *Completed balloon placement in the proximal descending aorta through a Teflon graft sutured to the ascending aorta. The graft is tunneled to a subcutaneous location in the subxiphoid region of the abdomen. Reprinted with permission from Krause AH, Bigelow JC, Page US. Transthoracic intraaortic balloon cannulation to avoid repeat sternotomy for removal. Ann Thorac Surg 1976;21:562–565.*

total of 23 patients undergoing transthoracic IABP placement.(17, 24) Meldrum-Hanna et al, reporting on a series of 8 patients who underwent transthoracic insertion via a vascular graft with the removal of the balloon percutaneously found fifty percent of patients had no complications at all.(53) The other complications consisted of 1 episode of mediastinitis

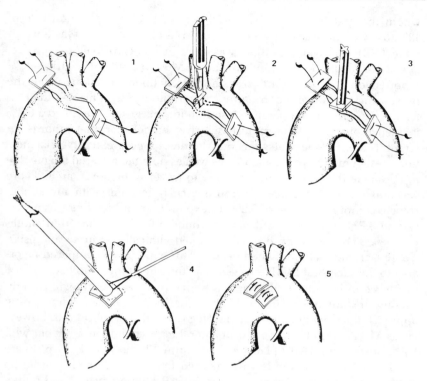

Figure 6.2. *Insertion of the balloon catheter through the aortic arch: (1) Two mattress sutures of O silk are placed, and Teflon pledget buttresses are spaced approximately 7 mm apart in a radial direction. (2) A stab wound is made in the aorta perpendicular to the mattress sutures. A No. 11 blade should be used, with penetration halfway up the bevel. (3) If it is necessary to dilate the stab wound, this is done first. The balloon catheter is then inserted into the incision. (4) After the balloon is inserted, the sutures are drawn through a rubber ligature tube and clamped to hold the balloon catheter in place. (5) After the procedure the catheter is removed and the mattress sutures are tied. Reprinted with permission from Shirkey AL, Loughridge BP, Lain KC. Insertion of the intraaortic balloon through the aortic arch. Ann Thorac Surg 1976;21:560–561.*

requiring later graft removal, and the inability to close the chest in one patient due to the presence of the balloon in the anterior mediastinum. Both of these patients survived. There were two deaths, one who suffered left main coronary artery embolization at the time of balloon removal, and one patient who had inadvertent cannulation of the axillary artery requiring IABP removal, with the patient later succumbing to intractable left ventricular failure. IABP-related mortality was 12.5%. Snow and Horrigan used transthoracic insertion as the method of choice in intra-operative cases, and reported only one transient neurologic deficit and no IABP-related mortality.(48) McGeehin et al reported on 39 patients in whom the graft technique was used, with a total complication rate of 13%.(54) Cerebrovascular accident occurred in 10%, which was unrelated to IABP removal, and there was a 5% incidence of balloon rupture, and 2.5% mediastinal wound infection. Most recently, Hazelrigg et al reported on a series of 100 transthoracic balloon insertions using the pursestring technique requiring repeat sternotomy.(49) This was the preferred method of intraoperative insertion for this group. He noted a 6.2% incidence of late balloon rupture, which is higher than that reported in femoral use. He speculates this may be due to more extensive calcification present in the proximal aorta, as well as possible material fatigue due to the angle the balloon must assume to traverse the aortic arch. There was only a 2.5% incidence of cerebrovascular accident, with a total neurologic complication rate of 6.2%. Reexploration for bleeding was necessary in 3.7% of patients, and sternal wound infection occurred in another 3.7%. There were no dissections noted clinically or in 15 autopsies. There were no balloon-related deaths. This experience compared favorably to their femoral IABP experience at the same time, who had a 16.3% incidence of vascular ischemia, and a total of 16.4% neurologic complications, including strokes in 12.2%. The use of an ascending aortic approach does not guarantee against leg ischemic complications, however, as Mackenzie et al reported unilateral leg ischemia in a patient who had transthoracic IABP placement performed because of known severe PVD.(32) Other authors have compared femoral and ascending aortic approaches. Macoviak et al, early on in IABP experience, found only a 4% complication rate with transaortic insertion as compared with 25% for femoral cannulation.(9) The complications in the transaortic group were a 4.2% occurrence of bowel ischemia, and 4.2% spinal ischemia. Another instance of bowel ischemia associated with ascending aortic insertion has also been reported, as has renal artery thrombosis.(58, 59) Pinkard and co-workers recently found no significant difference in wound problems in patients who had aortic vs femoral insertion, and a 28.4% incidence of leg complications in the femoral group vs none in the aortic cohort.(60) The mortality rate was higher in patients who had transthoracic insertion, but on multiple regression analysis the mode of insertion was not a predictor of operative death. Patients who underwent aortic insertion of the IABP were found to be more likely small and female, to have carotid bruits and more likely to have a prior history of stroke or cerebrovascular accident. Despite this apparent increased prevalence of risk factors for neurologic events, there was no statistically different incidence of neurologic complications compared with the femoral group. Naunheim et al also noted the association of transthoracic balloon insertion with increased mortality, but cited no specific complications of the technique, which would seem to implicate the impact of more significantly impaired cardiac function secondary to more extensive atherosclerosis.(39)

Therefore, although the initial impression that transaortic insertion of IABP is significantly more dangerous than conventional femoral insertion has not been proved in several studies, it must be remembered that the total number of patients in these reviews is still quite small, and expanding this mode of insertion to all patients requiring insertion of IABP during cardiac operation is probably unwarranted. However, the technique is of great utility in patients for whom there are difficulties with conventional insertion, and should be used whenever clinically indicated. Other novel methods of cannulation for IABP insertion, including subclavian and axillary artery have been used in situations where the femoral-iliac system cannot be cannulated, and there are contraindications to the use of the ascending aorta, such as multiple proximal anastomoses, aortotomy, or prohibitive atherosclerosis.(61) Axillary artery insertion has also been used for longer term balloon support as in a bridge to transplantation. (62) (Fig. 6.3)

Prevention and Treatment of Ischemia

Prevention of the vascular complications of IABP is obviously the best mode of treatment, but often hard to achieve in patients who very frequently have atherosclerotic peripheral vascular disease in addition to cardiac disease. The absence of PVD symptoms and the presence of normal pulses before insertion does not rule out the presence of clinical PVD, as seen in the study by Perler et al.(8) Of the patients who sustained vascular complications, 95% denied previous symptoms, and 75% had normal pulses, yet most were found to have severe disease at the time of open insertion. Careful examination of pulses and extremities should be performed in all patients before undergoing cardiac procedures, whether surgical or medical, to document the presence or absence of ischemia, and potentially note the "better" of the two limbs to be used for IABP insertion should the need arise. Aortography has been recommended as a pre-procedure diagnostic study in patients felt to be at high risk for balloon placement, but the study was not always successful at predicting the better side to use.(26) Report has also been made of the performance of angioplasty in the catheterization laboratory of a diseased iliac artery to allow for insertion of a balloon pump.(63) The determination of high risk for the need for IABP support is difficult and the risk factors some have found associated with IABP complications are of similarly low predictive value.(39) In addition, in today's medical economic and medicolegal climate, the performance of extensive invasive testing with low benefit is not a supportable concept. Noninvasive vascular laboratory testing may be a safer and more easily obtainable diagnostic test, but is again of low sensitivity and specificity for predicting complications, although Kvilekval et al noted all vascular complications to occur in patients with preoperative ankle/brachial indexes of < 0.6.(33) Preoperative vascular

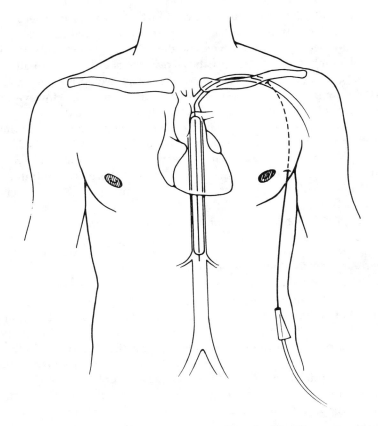

Figure 6.3. *Intra-aortic balloon pump positioned in the descending aorta. Reprinted with permission from McBride LR, Miller LW, Naunheim KS, Pennington DG. Axillary artery insertion of an intraaortic balloon pump. Ann Thorac Surg 1989;48:874–875.*

studies may be useful in planning the necessary reconstruction if vascular complications do occur, or in considering the risk-benefit ratio of a prophylactic IABP. Fortunately, the use of balloon pumps for prophylactic purposes seems to be decreasing. The fact that many balloon pumps need to be inserted emergently without the luxury of any pre-procedure assessment is a further complicating factor. In a patient with documented severe vascular disease undergoing an elective procedure, some type of "game plan" can be developed beforehand to address the possible contingencies, which could include planned open insertion of a femoral IABP, or possibly an ascending aortic approach at the time of cardiac surgery. In patients undergoing open heart surgery who seem to be at high risk for the need for a perioperative balloon pump, a guidewire, or arterial line can be placed in the groin preoperatively to aid in placement during weaning from bypass if it proves necessary. This approach would seem to provide for better success in cannulation and avoidance of some of the possible vascular injury that has been reported in patients who had poor pulses at the time of attempted insertion due to low flow states. The technique is obviously also readily applicable to the cardiac catheterization setting, where guidewire exchange to an IABP is usually a simple procedure. In most instances, however, the clinician must make a risk-benefit decision at the time based on whatever history is obtainable, and place the balloon by what seems to be the most reasonable technique into the better artery. Percutaneous insertion is still the appropriate first choice, except in patients who have had recently placed vascular grafts. The smallest possible balloon and sheath should be used, but the advantage to the wire-guided balloon, which is slightly larger than the non–wire-guided balloon, may outweigh the size difference, except in very small patients. Balloons designed for percutaneous insertion without an introducer sheath may be helpful in preventing complications in a patient with known vascular disease. Fluoroscopy may be useful in the insertion of patients with very tortuous arteries. The balloon is inserted with all possible care, with control of the temptation to push "just a little harder" when resistance is encountered. The option for a cut down if percutaneous insertion fails is the next step, but requires a surgeon to be readily available. If there is inability to cannulate either groin in a patient who remains unstable, urgent cardiac surgery must be considered if there is a surgically approachable lesion, and also allows for placement of the IABP via the ascending aorta, or by axillary or subclavian cannulation. Another recently available option is the use of another form of cardiac assistance such as temporary ventricular devices placed via an open chest, or potentially one of the more long-term devices.

Once the balloon is inserted, frequent, careful assessment of the limb must be performed by the nursing staff using the Doppler, if necessary. Most vascular complications will be evident at the time of insertion or within the first 24 hours after insertion.(29) Mild ischemia, consisting of only loss of pulses but with continued good vascular perfusion by evidence of capillary refill and/or the presence of Doppler signal, and without symptoms of ischemia, can be managed expectantly with continued careful observation and the removal of the IABP as soon as the patient will tolerate it hemodynamically. The first intervention in the treatment of the more severely ischemic limb is pullback or removal of the introducer sheath. If this does not provide adequate reversal of ischemia, the balloon should be removed. Balloon pumps placed percutaneously should be removed at the bedside, because this will often be adequate therapy for ischemia. Further surgical intervention is required in 30 to 50% of patients. Thrombectomy with local arterial repair is usually all that is needed, although more extensive reconstruction is necessary in some patients. If ischemia was untreated for a period of time, adjunctive fasciotomy may be needed to achieve limb salvage. Even if the IABP is removed successfully percutaneously in patients who are asymptomatic, or have recovery of perfusion with removal, the limbs must still be carefully followed up, because late thrombosis or embolism can occur.

Although the preferred treatment of severe limb ischemia is the removal of the IABP catheter, this may not be possible in patients who are very balloon dependent despite maximal pharmacologic support. Immediate removal is required for the classic indications of motor and sensory deficit in a patient who is responsive, or when there is objective evidence of severe ischemia in a sedated or unconscious patient in order to prevent the serious sequelae of unrecognized or untreated vascular insufficiency, including the need for fasciotomy, amputation, or development of motor or sensory deficits. Removal of the balloon and replacement in the contralateral femoral artery is a possibility, but atherosclerotic peripheral vascular disease is often symmetrical, so that the same vascular compromise may ultimately ensue. Placement into the ascending aorta as previously detailed is another option, but requires sternotomy. Another approach, first proposed by Barsamian et al in 1976, is the placement of a femerofemoral graft to provide improved inflow to the ischemic limb (64) (Fig. 6.4). The procedure has been reported with the use of Dacron, polytetrafluoroethylene (PTFE) or autogenous vein grafts. (64–67) Some surgeons have also divided between the insertion site of the balloon pump and the graft anastomosis to avoid the possibility for downstream embolism of thrombus at the time of IABP removal, or the potential for contamination of the fem-fem graft if open balloon removal is performed (65, 67) (Fig. 6.5). Several small series have reported the results this therapy. Gold et al performed X-femoral bypass in 10 patients and removed the grafts at the time of balloon removal in three women who had minimal atherosclerosis, but had small arteries that were obstructed by the balloon itself. (66) These patients had good long-term results without continued presence of the inflow graft. One patient required later graft removal for question of infection; one required fasciotomy for irreversible ischmia due to low flow, which ultimately led to death; and two patients, both of whom were older and had significant atherosclerosis, required later femoropopliteal reconstruction. Friedell et al followed up 28 of 29 long-term survivors of fem-fem bypass for balloon-related ischemia.(67) He did not routinely remove any grafts. At follow up forty-six percent of survivors were asymptomatic and 14% had mild claudication unchanged from their pre-existing PVD symptoms. Eighteen percent had sustained irreversible ischemic sequelae before grafting, and 7% developed infection, all of whom were operated on early in the series by open IABP insertion and removal technique. Since the advent of percutaneous balloons, no further infections have been noted. Fourteen per-

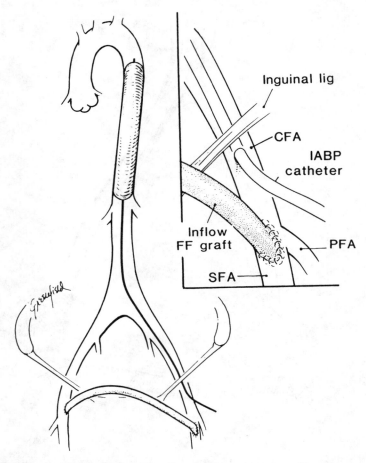

Figure 6.4. *Operative technique. Typical arrangement of patient with indwelling balloon catheter and femorofemoral bypass graft. Inset, Details of operative technique at site of distal outflow anastomosis and balloon catheter insertion site. Reprinted with permission from Gold JP, Cohen J, Shemin RJ et al. Femorofemoral bypass to relieve acute ischemia during intra-aortic balloon pump support. J Vasc Surg 1986;3:351–354.*

cent of patients developed new progressive claudication following the X-femoral graft. There was evidence of inflow vessel stenosis in three of the four patients, but because the symptoms were not severe, invasive studies preparatory to surgery were not performed, so that the exact etiology is unknown. Two of the four patients were young women found to have small arteries at the time of IABP insertion. Miller and co-workers emphasize the necessity of prompt revascularization as soon as severe ischemia is diagnosed in balloon-dependent patients, citing the need for

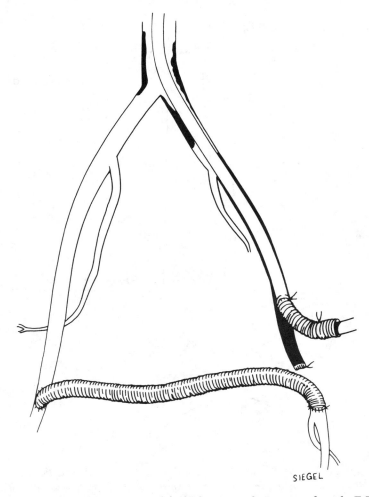

Figure 6.5. *Drawing of divided proximal femoral artery with separation from the F-F graft. Reprinted with permission from Alpert JA, Parsonnet V, Goldenkranz RJ et al. Limb ischemia during intra-aortic balloon pumping: Indication for femorofemoral crossover graft. J Thorac Cardiovasc Surg 1980;79:729–734.*

fasciotomy and amputation due to delayed revascularization in one third of the 11% of ischemic patients who required extra-anatomic bypass in his series.(35) Axillofemoral bypass has also been reported as a modality of improving inflow, but is much less common (35, 41) A final novel "solution" to the problem of severe ischemia in the balloon-dependent patient is proposed by Opie et al, who describes the successful reversal of ischemia in seven of eight patients who were treated with infusion of a dilute papaverine solution via the distal (central pressure) lumen of the

IABP, along with the addition of local therapy (warming lights, topical vasodilators).(68)

Long-Term Follow-Up

Despite all the literature on the acute consequences of intra-aortic balloon pump use, there is very little information on the long-term follow-up of patients who have undergone this procedure. Pace et al, in 1977, reported that 28% of hospital survivors had worsened arterial problems post discharge, of whom 18% required later reconstructive procedures.(7) On the other hand, Felix in 1981 found only 1 of 31 patients worse at follow up, who already had pre-existing PVD at the time of IABP insertion.(69) Kantrowitz et al reported only a 1% incidence of late vascular problems, requiring surgery in 62% of cases.(22) Alderman et al found a 10% incidence of late ischemia that was asymptomatic in more than 75% of patients.(29) Hedenmark and co-workers found poor relief of symptoms due to balloon pump related vascular complications in his series.(30) Of 18 patients who required surgical interventions, only two obtained long-term relief. At long-term follow-up, claudication was present in 17% of survivors. Funk et al conducted a study published in 1989 that found an overall incidence of vascular complications of 47%, 14% of which were major, most of these requiring surgical intervention.(70) These patients were then followed up for 12 to 20 months.(71) Unilateral ischemia was found in 18% of patients, and had worsened over time in 14% of patients. Eleven percent of patients had unilateral claudication and rest pain, whereas 8% had paresthesias and other neurologic symptoms. Five percent of patients who had been asymptomatic on hospital discharge had developed symptoms; 18% of those patients with minor symptoms at discharge had worsened, as had 38% of those patients who had sustained ischemic complications. On multivariate analysis, factors that were predictive of late ischemia were the occurrence of acute limb ischemia at the time of balloon pump use, smoking history, and cardiogenic shock as the indication for insertion. It seems necessary, therefore, to follow patients who have had balloon pumps long term in order to grasp the full impact of the potential complications.

Intra-aortic Balloon Pump Rupture and Entrapment

Although generally related to the presence of atherosclerotic disease, the complication of intra-aortic balloon pump perforation/rupture, with the attendant potential for subsequent entrapment, is different from the local vascular complications and dissections considered previously. The incidence of this complication is much smaller, and the first instance of balloon perforation was not reported until 1973 when Scheidt et al noted a case of balloon rupture complicated by massive gas embolism, which led to the demise of the patient.(72) After this, several reports of balloon perforation were published, but it was not until 1986 that Aru et al recorded a case of balloon rupture that caused balloon entrapment in the femoral artery that required operative removal.(73) Since then, many cases of balloon perforation with or without entrapment have been noted(74–86) and there is the suggestion recently that the incidence of this complication is increasing.(87) In a study published in 1986 surveying his initial 733 IABP insertions, Kantrowitz et al found a balloon rupture rate of only 1.6%.(22) Stahl et al, in 1988, and Sutter et al, in 1991, cited rates of 2.4 and 3.5%, respectively.(77, 78) Alvarez, in the *ASAIO Journal* in 1992, reported mean incidences of 9% in 1990, and 10.1% for 1991 (range, 2.9 to 17%) in a survey of the majority of patients undergoing IABP insertion in Australia during those years.(87) The incidence of perforation has been noted to be different with different manufacturers of the IABP catheter,(77, 87) but the exact etiology and implications of this finding are not yet clear. Whether the true incidence is increasing as markedly as Alvarez et al (87) suggests, or whether there is earlier recognition and more thorough reporting of the complication than had been done previously, may account in part for the increase. In our own institution, balloon rupture and entrapment is no longer considered a rare event, but has become a recognized complication of IABP use that is readily recognized and promptly treated by all the nursing and surgical staff; but we have not reported our incidence of this complication. Other factors that may be involved in its increasing occurrence are the widespread use of the percutaneous catheter and insertion by operators of varying skill, although the late perforation risk is not usually affected by the insertion technique. Although most reports have not shown mortality associated with this complication, Sutter et al reported two deaths in his series giving a 10.5% mortality rate for those suffering rupture, with Alvarez reporting three deaths for a 7.3% mortality rate.(77, 87)

Prompt recognition and treatment of this complication are essential for good outcome. Balloon rupture is most commonly recognized by the appearance of blood in the gas drive shaft, which was seen in 56% of the series of 19 patients studied by Sutter et al, and in almost all other reports of balloon rupture.(73–77, 81, 84–86, 88–90) The leak alarm on the IABP console may be the sole indicator of rupture in a much smaller number of patients (16%), and thus it may be much harder to ascertain the occurrence of perforation.(77, 79) In Sutter's series, two patients who had only the occurrence of the console alarm as the marker of the event had the balloon left in situ for a period of time after the alarm and suffered neurologic sequelae. In most cases, however, the leakage alarm on most IABP consoles is not sensitive enough to detect the minute gas leakage that may occur with microscopic perforations of the balloon membrane. Other reported premonitory signs of balloon rupture are the loss of pre-existing diastolic augmentation, and the need for frequent refilling of the system to offset this augmentation loss. The complication may also present as sudden onset of severe vascular ischemia due to vascular obstruction.(80) In a small number of patients, the balloon perforation is not recognized until the attempted removal of the IABP catheter when it is found to be entrapped as a consequence of clotted blood within the balloon lumen.(80, 82)

Perforation early after insertion is mainly due to mechanical or technical problems at the time of insertion. Sutter et al, in their article entitled "Events Associated with Rupture of Intra-Aortic Balloon Counterpulsation Devices," offered a thorough discussion of causes of early perforation.(77) Despite quality control, there may be manufacturing defects that are not detected until the time of clinical use. Lack of sufficient suction on the catheter before insertion may lead to trauma to the balloon as it is inserted through the introducer. Contact with instruments at the time of insertion may cause damage that is exacerbated by contact with the atherosclerotic aorta later. Attention must be paid to the angulation of the catheter and insertion sheath to avoid damage, particularly to the proximal junction of the balloon and the gas drive shaft. If the initial introduction of the needle into the artery approaches 90 degrees, the sheath and catheter must subsequently make a very sharp angle on entering the artery, which can lead to dislocation of the shaft from the balloon, as well as contact of the balloon membrane with the relatively sharp edge of the introducer or the central core of the balloon. This can lead to balloon membrane damage, or dislocation of the central core from the balloon itself. Similar problems with angulation can occur in obese individuals by traction on the soft tissues at the time of needle or introducer insertion. The small, atherosclerotic femoral artery can lacerate the balloon as it is first inserted, but this is usually rapidly recognized with blood seen in the balloon or catheter during insertion or at initial inflation of the IABP. The use of the available longer introducer sheath that extends past the femoral artery may be useful in preventing this problem with insertion. Difficulty in advancing the catheter over the wire suggests that the balloon is no longer following the intravascular path of the wire, or is impacted against an atherosclerotic plaque in the more proximal aorta, which can lead to membrane damage, or vascular perforation.

Although the numbers are small, some factors have been noted to be associated with IABP rupture. Stahl et al found an association between a history of hypertension and balloon rupture in his series of nine patients.(78) In addition, a predictive factor in his patients was the significantly higher diastolic augmentation that occurred in patients who suffered balloon rupture compared with control patients (Fig. 6.6). Higher diastolic augmentation is associated with a greater degree of coaptation of the balloon surface with the aorta(91), leading to the potential for

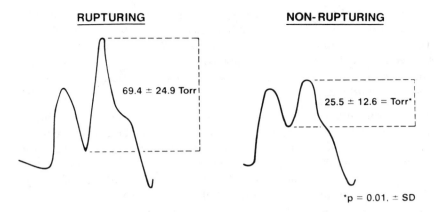

RUPTURING   **NON-RUPTURING**

69.4 ± 24.9 Torr

25.5 ± 12.6 = Torr*

*p = 0.01, ± SD

Figure 6.6. *Diastolic augmentation in rupturing and nonrupturing intra-aortic balloons. Note that diastolic augmentation was 2.5 times greater in patients with rupturing
balloons than in patients with nonrupturing devices. Reprinted with permission from Stahl
KD, Tortolani AJ, Nelson RL et al. Intraaortic balloon rupture. ASAIO Transactions
1988;34:496–499.*

increased contact with atherosclerotic plaques and thus abrasion and perforation of the balloon material, which is the predominant etiology of balloon perforations occurring late after insertion. The eccentricity of the
plaques can also cause asymmetrical stress on the balloon leading to membrane fatigue and increased predisposition to perforation. Microscopic
examination of balloons that ruptured late after insertion showed evidence of abrasion at the site of perforation and at other sites on the balloon.(22, 77–79, 81, 88) Further evidence for the abrasion/perforation
theory is that several patients have been reported to have perforated one
or more balloons at approximately the same site.(77, 81) The perforations
also tend to occur in the more proximal portion of femorally inserted balloons where the diameter of the distal abdominal aorta is smaller and also
more likely to be diseased allowing for more contact of the IABP membrane with calcified plaque.

The major complications associated with IABP rupture are vascular
entrapment and gas embolism. Additionally, there can be a period of low
cardiac output during the time the balloon is being changed if the patient
is balloon dependent, but this is not commonly a cause of significant
morbidity. Balloon entrapment, particularly when not suspected due to a
lack of blood in the catheter or other signs of perforation, can be a serious complication and has led to death secondary to vascular injury.
Potentially due to the slow process of the microscopic leak before blood
is detected in the tubing, or the high thrombogenicity of the interior of
the balloon, extremely hard clots can be found in the balloon that

obstruct, particularly if the procedure is attempted percutaneously. Too vigorous traction has been known to result in "eversion endarterctomy" of vascular segments or total avulsion of distal vessels even under direct vision of the insertion site.(80, 84) Appropriate measures to remove the device include exposing the site of balloon insertion, careful extraction of as much of the catheter as can be removed without undue force, and the localization and exposure of the site of the balloon entrapment. Millham et al underlined the utility of a flat plate abdominal film taken in the operating room in order to discern the level of entrapment.(80) Adequate exposure for proximal and distal arterial control can then be judiciously planned out. Sometimes, the site of entrapment is in the common femoral artery, which requires only division of the inguinal ligament, but exposure of the entire distal aorta may be necessary via an abdominal or retroperitoneal approach. (80, 82) There are two reports of the use of a thrombolytic agent, streptokinase or tissue plasminogen activator, injected via the gas drive line of the catheter to dissolve the clot to allow for safe percutaneous removal.(75, 84) In cases in which the loss of balloon support causes hemodynamic instability, or catastrophic vascular compromise, however, there appears to be no alternative to prompt, careful surgical removal by direct arterial exposure and removal at the site of entrapment.

Gas embolism with neurologic injury is the other most significant complication of balloon perforation, but is fortunately very rare, even in patients who have sustained balloon rupture. Three cases of fatal gas embolism have been reported, (17, 72, 92) but these were all due to direct trauma to the balloon at the time of insertion. A nonfatal but significant embolus causing persistent neurologic deficit has been reported due to fracture of the central lumen of a balloon catheter that released a presumably large volume of gas before detection.(93) Helium is used as the driving gas because of its low weight and therefore good distensibility characteristics especially in the presence of tachycardia. It is less soluble in blood than carbon dioxide, however, and Furman and co-workers have shown 20 to 40 cc boluses of helium to be rapidly fatal in an animal model.(94) It is felt that the low incidence of neurological sequelae in most instances is due to the microscopic size of the usual balloon perforation and the low pressure, even during maximum balloon inflation. The low pressure in the balloon during inflation and the negative pressure during deflation allows blood to enter the balloon and give evidence of the perforation before sufficient gas has escaped to cause injury. This is supported by the finding that Sutter's two patients who sustained neurologic injury did not have prompt recognition of the balloon rupture and the catheters were left in for a rather prolonged period of time possibly allowing gas egress before the diagnosis was made and the balloon removed.(77) Frederikson et al reported a case of a patient who suffered helium embolism from a ruptured IABP and was treated in a hyperbaric chamber with good resolution of the neurologic deficits, but this is not an option available to most practitioners due to the small number of hyperbaric chambers available for clinical use.(95)

Other Complications

Paraplegia

Since Tyras et al first report of paraplegia following the use of an IABP in 1978, there have been a total of 13 cases of this complication in the literature.(9, 96–104) Macoviak et al reported three cases in a series of 178 patients, for an incidence of 1.7%.(9) Almost all of the other citations are of single cases that would suggest a similarly low incidence.(96–103) All of the balloon pumps involved were inserted femorally, except for one that was transaortic.(9) Almost all of the cases occurred late after balloon pump insertion, including one patient who did not develop the complication until 3 days after the balloon pump was removed.(99) Six of the thirteen patients died, most of multisystem organ failure, for an associated mortality rate of 46%. Tyras reported a subadventitial hematoma with intact aortic intima at the level of the spinal arteries,(96) and there were two other probable dissections although this diagnosis was not proved on any diagnostic study.(99, 101) Autopsy showed one definite occlusion of the spinal arteries by atheroemboli that had also affected other organs.(100) Unfortunately, although the presumption was that atheroemboli were responsible, no definite etiology was ever able to be determined in the other cases.(102, 103) Because diffuse atherosclerosis is a common occurrence in patients who have significant cardiovascular disease, the prevention or avoidance of this complication is therefore extremely difficult.

Arterial Compromise of Other Vessels

Although arterial dissection or shower of atherosclerotic emboli can compromise the entire distal aortic run-off, there have been several cases of discrete organ injury due to IABP, most often due to malposition of the balloon. In abnormally distal placement of femoral balloon catheters, occlusion and/or injury to the left subclavian and carotid artery have been reported.(105, 106) In one of these cases, occlusion of the left subclavian artery led to the discard of a left internal artery mammary graft that had been prepared for grafting, but was found to have poor flow.(106) The etiology of this difficulty was not determined until the postoperative period. Insertion of the balloon pump through the ascending aorta does not obviate the risk of catheter tip malposition. In one patient, a catheter tip impacted in the superior mesenteric artery caused near total small bowel infarction, which led to the patient's demise.(58) Comment is made in the report that it is known from vascular radiology experience how easy it is to cannulate the anteriorly placed abdominal arteries from above. The author points out that a flat plate alone is not sufficient to confirm position of the tip of an ascending aortic balloon. Particularly in a patient who is having abdominal pain, a lateral abdominal film should be obtained to check the position of the catheter tip. Pace et al, in 1977, had reported two cases of bowel ischemia related to IABP use that caused death, but the type of cannulation is unspecified.(7) A case of renal artery thrombosis occurred after an ascending balloon catheter was removed whose tip had been at the level of the renal artery orifices.(59) Presumably, a thrombus that had been on the catheter tip was dislodged into the renal arteries at the time of balloon removal, possibly echoing the complication Scheidt and co-workers reported in 1973 of "renal embolus."(72) Mesenteric and left renal artery thrombosis was reported after removal of a conventionally placed femoral IABP.(35) Atheroemboli secondary to IABP function have also caused organ injury. Harris et al reported a case of multiple organ involvement, including spinal cord, and Busch discrete splenic infarction from cholesterol emboli. (100, 107)

Infection

The open femoral technique with prosthetic vascular graft used in the early IABP experience was associated with a 3 to 5% incidence of local wound problems. Some of these could be effectively treated with only local debridement, dressing changes, and antibiotics, but others were associated with sepsis and death, or required later removal of prosthetic material, some with the need for extra-anatomic reconstruction.(2, 5, 8, 10) The incidence of infection has decreased markedly with the current widespread use of the percutaneous catheter. In the most recent experience local infection is rarely noted, with only one case occurring for an incidence of 1.3% in one series.(34) Most other recent reports of infection or sepsis involve the open placement of percutaneous catheters. (31, 35) In patients who had IABP assistance for a prolonged period of time as bridge to transplantation (mean, 11.3 days; range, 5 to 46 days), Lazar et al did report a 13% incidence of infection.(108) Contrary to previous reports that showed the relationship of increased infection to longer balloon duration, he found no increase in the rate of infection after the first 5 days of therapy, suggesting the introduction of infection at the time of insertion. The presence of diabetes does impact on the incidence of infection. In a group of diabetic patients, 13% who had percutaneous insertion and the rest open, Wasfie noted the occurrence of infectious complications in 37% of insulin-dependent diabetics, 22% in those with NIDDM, and 25% of nondiabetic patients, showing the influence of altered white cell function and peripheral vascular disease contributing to the risk of infection in diabetics.(25)

Hematologic Effects

Ever since its introduction, it was noted that a modest thrombocytopenia developed in many patients who had balloon pump therapy.(2, 3) Many of the patients who had thrombocytopenia associated with IABP use also had concurrent cardiac surgery that is known to cause thrombocytopenia on its own; therefore, separating out the influence of the balloon pump alone is difficult. Nevertheless, the degree of thrombocytopenia potentially occurring with IABP use is not of any clinical significance.(8,15) Because of the pulsation of the balloon and the interaction with the surrounding blood, another early concern was of the potential for hemolysis secondary to the pulsation of the balloon, which also has not proved to be a problem.(8) Although some studies do cite the need for blood transfusion in IABP patients, this has most often been related to catheter site bleeding, other vascular complications or to the critical illness itself rather than a significant hemolytic anemia.(23)

Delirium

Delirium is a complication of major illness reported to occur in approximately 10% of hospitalized patients.(109) A recent study has documented a rate of occurrence of delirium in 34% of balloon-dependent patients who required significant psychotropic medication for control.(110) The patients who suffered delirium were older, with a more frequent history of seizures and organic brain syndrome than those who did not experience delirium. Although there was no higher mortality rate associated with delirium, the hospital stay was significantly longer for the affected patients, and there was a much higher incidence of residual organic brain syndrome in the affected patients. Delirium is thought to be caused by dysfunction in the acetylcholine and dopaminergic neurotransmitter system that can be affected by cardiovascular disorders. The periods of brain hypoperfusion associated with low cardiac output states and while the patients are undergoing IABP therapy may exacerbate this defect. In addition, ICU patients not infrequently develop psychiatric disorders due to the conditions found in an ICU. Treatment of delirium in the IABP patients was most effectively and safely treated with high doses of intravenous haloperidol, which has minimal effects on cardiac and respiratory function.

Conclusion

In summary, the intra-aortic balloon counterpulsation device is an extremely useful tool in the treatment of cardiac disease. Insertion is able to be achieved percutaneously in greater than 90 to 95% of patients. Its use is not without risks, however. The most common complication of IABP use is vascular ischemia, generally occurring in 5 to 20% of patients, with the need for surgical correction in one third to one half of these cases. Fortunately, the development of the wire-guided balloon pump has nearly eliminated the catastrophic and deadly problems of aortic dissection and perforation. Percutaneous insertion has also virtually eliminated infection as a complication of use, and all other complications including paraplegia, balloon rupture and entrapment, and mesenteric ischemia, fortunately, are rare. Factors that have been found to be associated with morbidity in many studies are female gender and the presence of underlying peripheral vascular disease. Obesity and other factors co-morbid with peripheral vascular disease, such as diabetes and smoking history, may also be risk factors. Percutaneous insertion does have a higher risk of associated vascular complications than open surgical insertion, but if performed carefully, the risk-benefit ratio seems favorable for its use. Longer duration of support does not seem to contribute significantly to morbidity. No combination of risk factors is a strong predictor of morbidity, however, and problems can occur in patients without any seeming predisposition to complications, and do not happen in patients who seem to be at high risk. The occurrence of vascular complications, however, does not appear to contribute significantly to overall mortality, which seems rather to be determined by overall cardiovascular reserve. The complications can be serious sources of morbidity, and the clinician must be able to recognize and provide for the appropriate treatment in order to achieve the best results. Long-term follow-up is necessary to appreciate the full extent of the complications of IABP use.

REFERENCES

1. Allpert J, Bhaktan EK, Gielchinsky L et al. Vascular Complications of intra-aortic balloon pumping. Arch Surg 1976;111:1190–1195.
2. McCabe JC, Abel RM, Subramanian VA, Gay, WA. Complications of Intra-aortic balloon insertion and counterpulsation. Circ 1978;57:769–773.
3. Weber KT, Janicki JS. Intraaortic balloon counterpulsation. A review of physiological principles, clinical results, and device safety. Ann Thorac Surg 1974; 17:602–636.
4. Lefemine AA, Kosowsky B, Madoff I, Black H, Lewis M. Results and complications of intraaortic balloon pumping in surgical and medical patients. Am J Cardiol 1977;40:416–420.
5. McEnany MT, Kay HR, Buckley MJ, et al. Clinical experience with intraaortic balloon pump support in 728 patients. Circ 1978;58:(suppl 1, no. 3) I:124–132.
6. Golding LAR, Loop FD, Peter M, Cosgrove DM, Taylor PC, Phillips DF. Late survival following use of intraaortic balloon pump in revascularization operations. Ann Thorac Surg 1980;30:48–51.
7. Pace PD, Tilney NL, Lesch M, Couch NP. Peripheral arterial complications of intra-aortic balloon counterpulsation. Surgery 1977;82:685–688.
8. Perler BA, McCabe CJ, Abbott WM, Buckley MJ. Vascular complications of intra-aortic balloon counterpulsation. Arch Surg 1983;118:957–962.
9. Macoviak J, Stephenson LW, Edmunds LH, Harken A, McVaugh H. The intra-aortic balloon pump: An analysis of five years experience. Ann Thorac Surg 1980;29:451–458.

10. Beckman CB, Geha AS, Hammond GL, Baue AE. Results and complications of intraaortic balloon counterpulsation. Ann Thorac Surg 1977;24:550–559.

11. Isner JM, Cohen SR, Virmani R, Lawrinson W, Roberts WC. Complications of the intraaortic balloon counterpulsation device: Clinical and morphologic observations in 45 necropsy patients. Am J Cardiol 1980;45:260–268.

12. Biddle TL, Stewart S, Stuard ID. Dissection of the aorta complicating intra-aortic balloon counterpulsation. Am Heart J 1976;6:781–784.

13. Bregman D, Casarella WJ. Percutaneous intraaortic balloon pumping: Initial clinical experience. Ann Thorac Surg 1980;29:153–155.

14. Bregman D, Nichols AB, Weiss MB, Powers ER, Martin EC, Casarella WJ. Percutaneous intraaortic balloon insertion. Am J Cardiol 1980;46:261–264.

15. Subramanian VA, Goldstein JE, Sos TA, McCabe JC, Hoover EA, Gay WA. Preliminary clinical experience with intraaortic balloon pumping. Circ 1980;62(suppl I):I:123–129.

16. Goldman BS, Hill TJ, Rosenthal GA, Scully HE, Weisel RD, Baird RJ. Complications associated with use of the intra-aortic balloon pump. Can J Surg 1982;25:153–156.

17. Pennington DG, Swartz M, Codd JE, Merjavy JP, Kaiser GC. Intraaortic balloon pumping in cardiac surgical patients: A nine year experience. Ann Thorac Surg 1983;36:125–131.

18. Shahian DM, Neptune WB, Ellis FH, Maggs PR. Intraaortic balloon pump morbidity: A comparative analysis of risk factors between percutaneous and surgical techniques. Ann Thorac Surg 1983;36:644–653.

19. Gottlieb SO, Brinker JA, Borkon AM, et al. Identification of patients at high risk for complications of intraaortic balloon counterpulsation: A multivariate risk factor analysis. Am J Cardiol 1984;53:1135–1139.

20. Iverson LIG, Herfindahl G, Ecker RR et al. Vascular complications of intraaortic balloon counterpulsation. Am J Surg 1987;154:99–103.

21. Curtis JJ, Boland M, Bliss D, et al. Intra-aortic balloon cardiac assist: Complication rates for the surgical and percutaneous insertion techniques. Am Surgeon 1988;54:142–147.

22. Kantrowitz A, Wasfie T, Freed PS, Rubenfire M, Wajszczuk, Schork MA. Intraaortic balloon pumping 1967-1982: Analysis of complications in 733 patients. Am J Cardiol 1986;57:976–983.

23. Goldberg MJ, Rubenfire M, Kantrowitz A, et al. Intraaortic balloon pump insertion: A randomized study comparing percutaneous and surgical techniques. J Am Coll Cardiol 1987;9:515–523.

24. Pelletier LC, Pomar JL, Bosch X, Galinanes M, Hebert Y. Complications of circulatory assistance with intra-aortic balloon pumping: A comparison of surgical and percutaneous techniques. J Heart Transplant 1986;5:138–142.

25. Wasfie T, Freed PS, Rubenfire M, et al. Risks associated with intraaortic balloon pumping in patients with and without diabetes mellitus. Am J Cardiol 1988;61:558–562.

26. Vignola PA, Swaye PS, Gosselin AJ. Guidelines for effective and safe percutaneous intraaortic balloon pump insertion and removal. Am J Cardiol 1981;48:660–664.

27. Cutler BS, Okike ON, Vander Salm TJ. Surgical versus percutaneous removal of the intra-aortic balloon. J Thorac Cardiovasc Surg 1983;86:907–911.

28. Leinbach RC, Goldstein J, Gold HK, Moses JW, Collins MB, Subramanian V. Percutaneous wire-guided balloon pumping. Am J Cardiol 1982;49: 1707–1710.

29. Alderman JD, Gabliani GI, McCabe CH, et al. Incidence and management of limb ischemia with percutaneous wire-guided intraaortic balloon catheters. Am Coll Cardiol 1987;9:524–530.

30. Hedenmark J, Ahn H, Henze A, Nystrom SO, Svedjeholm, Tyden H. Complications of intra-aortic balloon counterpulsation with special reference to limb ischemia. Scand J Thor Cardiovasc Surg 1988;22:123–125.

31. Eltchaninoff H, Dimas AP, Whitlow PL. Complications associated with percutaneous placement and use of intraaortic balloon counterpulsation. Am J Cardiol 1993;71:328–332.

32. Mackenzie DJ, Wagner WH, Kulber DA, et al. Vascular complications of the intra-aortic balloon pump. Am J Surg 1992;164:517–521.

33. Kvilekval KHV, Mason RA, Newton GB, Anagnostolpoulos CE, Vlay SC, Giron F. Complications of percutaneous intra-aortic balloon pump use in patients with peripheral vascular disease. Arch Surg 1991;126:621–623.

34. Yuen JC. Percutaneous intra-aortic balloon pump: Emphasis on complications. South Med J 1991;84:956–960.

35. Miller JS, Dodson TF, Salam AA, Smith RB. Vascular complications following intra-aortic balloon pump insertion. Am Surg 1992;58:233–238.

36. Phillips SJ, Tannenbaum M, Zeff RH, Iannone LA, Ghali M, Kongtahworn C. Sheathless insertion of the percutaneous intraaortic balloon pump: An alternate method. Ann Thorac Surg 1992;53:162.

37. Tatar H, Cicek S, Demirkilic U et al. Vascular complications of intraaortic balloon pumping: Unsheathed versus sheathed insertion. Ann Thorac Surg 1993;55:1518–1522.

38. Nash IS, Lorell BH, Fishman RF, Baim DS, Donahue C, Diver DJ. A new technique for sheathless percutaneous intraaortic balloon catheter insertion. Cath and Cardiovasc Diagnosis 1991;23:57–60.

39. Naunheim KS, Swartz MT, Pennington DG, et al. Intraaortic balloon pumping in patients requiring cardiac operations. Risk analysis and long-term follow-up. J Thorac Cardiovasc Surg 1992;104:1654–1661.

40. Barnett MG, Swartz MT, Peterson GJ, et al. Vascular complications from intraaortic balloons: Risk analysis. J Vasc Surg 1994;19:81–89.

41. Makhoul RG, Cole CW, McCann RL. Vascular complications of the intra-aortic balloon pump: An analysis of 436 patients. Am Surg 1993;59:564–568.

42. Alle KM, White GH, Harris JP, May J, Baird D. Iatrogenic vascular trauma associated with intra-aortic balloon pumping: Identification of risk factors. Am Surg 1993;59:813–817.

43. Mohr LL, Smith DC, Schaner GJ. Catheterization of synthetic vascular grafts. J Vasc Surg 1986;3:854–856.

44. Shahian DM, Jewell ER. Intraaortic balloon pump placement through Dacron aortofemoral grafts. J Vasc Surg 1988;7:795–797.

45. Burns RJ, Feindel CM. Intraaortic balloon pump placement through Dacron aortofemoral grafts. J Vasc Surg 1989;9:401.

46. LaMuraglia GM, Vlahakes GJ, Moncure AC, et al. The safety of intraaortic balloon pump catheter insertion through suprainguinal prosthetic vascular bypass grafts. J Vasc Surg 1991;13:830–837.

47. Gueldner TL, Lawrence GH. Intraaortic balloon assist through cannulation of the ascending aorta. Ann Thorac Surg 1975;19:88–91.

48. Snow N, Horrigan TP. Intraaortic balloon counterpulsation via the ascending aorta. J Cardiovasc Surg 1986;27:337–340.

49. Hazelrigg SR, Auer JE, Seifert PE. Experience in 100 transthoracic balloon pumps. Ann Thorac Surg 1992;54:528–532.

50. Krause AH, Bigelow JC, Page US. Transthoracic intraaortic balloon cannulation to avoid repeat sternotomy for removal. Ann Thorac Surg 1976;21:562–565.

51. Roe BB, Chatterjee K. Transaortic cannulation for balloon pumping: Report of a patient undergoing closed chest decannulation. Ann Thorac Surg 1976;21:568–570.

52. Nunez L, Aguado MG, Iglesias A, Larrea JL. Transaortic cannulation for balloon pumping in a "crowded aorta". Ann Thorac Surg 1980;30:400–402.

53. Meldrum-Hanna WG, Deal CW, Ross DE. Complications of ascending aortic intraaortic balloon pump cannulation. Ann Thorac Surg 1985;40:241–244.

54. McGeehin W, Sheikh F, Donahoo JS, Lechman MJ, MacVaugh H. Transthoracic intraaortic balloon pump support: Experience in 39 patients. Ann Thorac Surg 1987;44:26–30.

55. Bonchek LI, Olinger GN. Direct ascending aortic insertion of the "percutaneous" intraaortic balloon catheter in the open chest: Advantages and disadvantages. Ann Thorac Surg 1981;32:512–514.

56. Shirkey AL, Loughridge BP, Lain KC. Insertion of the intraaortic balloon through the aortic arch. Ann Thorac Surg 1976;21:560–561.

57. Phillips SJ, Zeff RH, Skinner JR. Cannulation of ascending aorta for IABP assist. Ann Thorac Surg 1986;41:583.

58. Jarmolowski CR, Poirer RL. Small bowel infarction complicating intra-aortic balloon counterpulsation via the ascending aorta. J Thorac Cardiovasc Surg 1980;79:735–737.

59. Baciewicz FA, Kaplan BM, Murphy TE, Neiman HL. Bilateral renal artery thrombotic occlusion: A unique complication following removal of a transthoracic intraaortic balloon. Ann Thorac Surg 1982;33:631–634.

60. Pinkhard J, Utley JR, Leyland SA, Morgan M, Johnson H. Relative risk of aortic and femoral insertion of intraaortic balloon pump after coronary artery bypass grafting procedures. J Thorac Cardiovasc Surg 1993;105:721–728.

61. Mayer JH. Subclavian artery approach for insertion of intra-aortic balloon. J Thorac Cardiovasc Surg 1978;76:61–63.

62. McBride LR, Miller LW, Naunheim KS, Pennington DG. Axillary artery insertion of an intraaortic balloon pump. Ann Thorac Surg 1989;48:874–875.

63. Cohn LH. Limb ischemia induced by intraaortic balloon pumping. J Thorac Cardiovasc Surg 1990;99:566.

64. Barsamian EM, Goldman M, Crane C, et al. Femorofemoral bypass graft in intra-aortic balloon counterpulsation. Arch Surg 1976;111:1070–1072.

65. Alpert JA, Parsonnet V, Goldenkranz RJ, et al. Limb ischemia during intra-aortic balloon pumping: Indication for femorofemoral crossover graft. J Thorac Cardiovasc Surg 1980;79:729–734.

66. Gold JP, Cohen J, Shemin RJ, et al. Femorofemoral bypass to relieve acute left ischemia during intra-aortic balloon pump cardiac support. J Vasc Surg 1986;3:351–354.
67. Friedell ML, Alpert J, Parsonnet V, et al. Femorofemoral grafts for lower limb ischemia caused by intra-aortic balloon pump. J Vasc Surg 1987;5:180–186.
68. Opie JC, Zavitzanos J, Bell-Thompson J. A simple "solution" worth consideration to combat limb ischemia induced by intraaortic balloon pumping. J Thorac Cardiovasc Surg 1989;98:295–296.
69. Felix WR, Barsamian E, Silverman AB. Long-term follow-up of limbs after the use of intra-aortic balloon counterpulsation device. Surgery 1982;91:183–187.
70. Funk M, Gleason J, Foell D. Lower limb ischemia related to use of the intraaortic balloon pump. Heart Lung 1989;18:542–552.
71. Funk M, Ford CF, Foell DW et al. Frequency of long-term lower limb ischemia associated with intraaortic balloon pump use. Am J Cardiol 1992;70:1195–1199.
72. Scheidt S, Willner G, Mueller H et al. Intraaortic balloon counterpulsation in cardiogenic shock: Report of a co-operative clinical trial. N Engl J Med 1973;288:979–984.
73. Aru GM, King JT, Hovaguimian H, Floten HS, Ahmad A, Starr A. The entrapped balloon: Report of a possibly serious condition. J Thorac Cardiovasc Surg 1986;91:146–149.
74. Milgalter E, Mosseri M, Uretzky G, Romanoff H. Intraaortic balloon entrapment: A complication of balloon perforation. Ann Thorac Surg 1986; 42:697–698.
75. Lambert CJ. Intraaortic balloon entrapment. Ann Thorac Surg 1987;44:446.
76. Brodell GK, Tuzcu EM, Weiss SJ, Simpfendorfer C. Intra-aortic balloon pump rupture and entrapment. Clev Clin J Med 1989;56:740–742.
77. Sutter FP, Joyce DH, Bailey BM et al. Events associated with rupture of intra-aortic balloon counterpulsation devices. ASAIO Transactions 1991;37:38–40.
78. Stahl KD, Tortolani AJ, Nelson RL et al. Intraaortic balloon rupture. ASAIO Transactions 1988;34:496–499.
79. Nishizawa J, Konishi Y, Matsumoto M, Yuasa S. Intraaortic balloon entrapment: A case report and a review of the literature. Jpn Circ J 1991;55:563–565.
80. Millham FH, Hudson HM, Woodson J, Menzoian JO. Intraaortic balloon pump entrapment. Ann Vasc Surg 1991;5:381.
81. Price C, Briffa NP, Lynn MAJ. Perforation of an intraaortic balloon twice in one patient. J Cardiovasc Surg 1992;33:44–45.
82. Olearchyk AS. Retained intraaortic balloon assist device. J Thorac Cardiovasc Surg 1992 103:1231–1232.
83. Alvarez JM, Brady PW, Wilson RM. Intra-aortic balloon rupture causing femoral entrapment. Aust NZ J Surg 1992;63:72–74.
84. Horowitz MD, Otero M, deMarchena EJ, Neibart RM, Novak S, Bolooki H. Intraaortic balloon entrapment. Ann Thorac Surg 1993;56:370–372.
85. Kolvekar S, Griffin S, Fisher A, O'Riordan J. Retained intraaortic balloon. Ann Thorac Surg 1993;55:1598–1599.
86. Shafei H, Al-Ebrahim K. Awareness of a serious complication of the intraaortic balloon pump: "Entrapping". Ann Thorac Surg 1994;57:1373.

87. Alvarez JM, Brady PW, McWilson R. Intra-aortic balloon rupture: An increasing trend? ASAIO Journal 1992;38:862–863.
88. Rajani R, Keon WJ, Bedard P. Rupture of an intraaortic balloon. J Thorac Cardiovasc Surg 1980;79:301–302.
89. Mayerhofer KE, Billhardt RA, Codini MA. Delayed abrasion perforation of two intra-aortic balloons. Am Heart J 1984;108:1361–1363.
90. Kayser KL. Abrasion perforation of intra-aortic balloons. Am Heart J.
91. Weber KT, Janicki JS, Walker AA. Intra-aortic pumping: An analysis of several variables affecting balloon performance. Trans Am Soc Artif Intern Organs 1972;27:486–491.
92. Finegan BA. Operative intra-aortic balloon rupture. Can J Anaesth 1988;35:297–299.
93. Myers GJ, Landymore RW, Leadon RB, Squires C. Fracture of the internal lumen of a Datascope Percor Stat-DL balloon, resulting in stroke. Ann Thorac Surg 1994;57:1335–1337.
94. Furman S, Vijaynagar R, Rosenbaum R et al. Lethal sequelae of intraaortic balloon rupture. Surgery 1971;69:121–129.
95. Frederickson JW, Smith J, Brown PUMP, Zinetti C. Arterial helium embolism from a ruptured intraaortic balloon. Ann Thorac Surg 1988; 46:690–692.
96. Tyras DH, Willman VL. Paraplegia following intraaortic balloon assistance. Ann Thorac Surg 1978;25:164–166.
97. Criado A, Agosti J, Horno R, Jiminez C. Paraplegia following balloon assistance after cardiac surgery. Scand J Thor Cardiovasc Surg 1981;15:103–104.
98. Rose DM, Jacobowitz IJ, Acinapura AJ, Cunningham JN. Paraplegia following percutaneous insertion of an intra-aortic balloon. J Thorac Cardiovasc Surg 1984;87:788–789.
99. Scott IR, Goiti JJ. Late paraplegia as a consequence of intraaortic balloon pump support. Ann Thorac Surg 1985;40:300–301.
100. Harris RE, Reimer KA, Crain BJ, Becsey DD, Oldham HN. Spinal cord infarction following intraaortic balloon support. Ann Thorac Surg 1986;42:206–207.
101. Seifert PE, Silverman NA. Late paraplegia resulting from intraaortic balloon pump. Ann Thorac Surg 1986;41:700.
102. Orr E, McKittrick J, D'Agostino R et al. Paraplegia following intra-aortic balloon support. J Cardiovasc Surg 1989;30:1013–1014.
103. Riggle KP, Oddi MA. Spinal cord necrosis and paraplegia as complications of the intra-aortic balloon. Crit Care Med 1989;17:475–476.
104. Singh BM, Fass AE, Pooley RW, et al. Paraplegia associated with intraaortic balloon pump counterpulsation. Stroke 1983;14:1983.
105. O'Rourke MF, Shepherd KM. Protection of the aortic arch and subclavian artery during intra-aortic balloon pumping. J Thorac Cardiovasc Surg 1973;65:543–546.
106. Rodigas PC, Bridges KG. Occlusion of left internal mammary artery with intra-aortic balloon: Clinical implications. J Thorac Cardiovasc Surg 1986;91:142–143.
107. Busch HM, Cogbill TH, Gunderson AE. Splenic infarction: Complication of intra-aortic balloon counterpulsation. Am Heart J 1985;109:383–385.

108. Lazar JM, Ziady GM, Dummer SJ, Thompson M, Ruffner RJ. Outcome and complications of prolonged intraaortic balloon counterpulsation in cardiac patients. Am J Cardiol 1992;69:955–958.
109. Lipowski ZJ. Delirium (acute confusional states). JAMA 1987;258:1789–1792.
110. Sanders KM, Stern TA, O'Gara PT et al. Delirium during intra-aortic balloon pump therapy. Psychosomatics 1992;33:35–44.

7

Nursing Care of the Intra-aortic Balloon Pump Patient

Betty T. Sadaniantz

Nursing Care of the Intra-aortic Balloon Pump Patient

Introduction

The critical care nurse who has never cared for the intra-aortic balloon pump (IABP) patient may be initially intimidated by the equipment and a feeling of overwhelming responsibility for the patient. In fact, the IABP is a relatively simple machine in design and operation that provides modest circulatory support with minimal complications. It is the goal of this chapter to de-mystify the theory and practice of IABP counterpulsation for the clinical nurse.

The critical care nurse plays a pivotal role in the care of the patient treated with an IABP. Nursing assessment skills and knowledge of anatomy and pathophysiology will provide valuable information to assist the physician in making this treatment choice and managing the patient throughout the IABP treatment. Her intensive interactions with the patient and prompt interventions contribute immeasurably toward therapeutic management. In many facilities, the nurse has primary responsibility for balloon timing and augmentation and, therefore, must possess expertise in the operation of the console and invasive devices.

Acuity may easily approach 24 hours of required direct nursing care per day for a patient with an IABP. The clinical status is critical, changes occur rapidly, and nursing vigilance is required to safely manage patient care. Many nurses find the care of an IABP patient to be both exciting in its demands and rewarding because of the dramatic recoveries and beneficial effects.

Patients treated with IABPs are always managed in critical care areas, such as a medical intensive care unit, surgical intensive care unit, or a coronary care unit. The intra-aortic balloon catheter may be placed in the operating room, cardiac catheterization laboratory, emergency unit, special procedure area, or at the patient's bedside, depending on the facility's physical space, available resources, and policies and procedures. For the purposes of this chapter, it is assumed that the patient will be maintained in the critical care unit.

Indications for Intra-aortic Balloon Pumping

The nurse is in a unique position, by virtue of close and extended contact with patients, to recognize those situations that may benefit from intra-aortic balloon augmentation through the stabilization of patient hemodynamics. These include those conditions in which it would be desirable to enhance cardiac output, decrease afterload, and increase coronary artery perfusion. Use of the IABP may help relieve intractable ischemic chest pain and limit myocardial infarct size. A list of common indications for the IABP is presented in Table 7.1.(1–8)

The best results of IABP therapy are obtained when there are reversible conditions, such as myocardial ischemia, stunned or hibernating myocardium, or when the presenting problem can ultimately be corrected surgically, such as mitral valve incompetence, true left ventricular aneurysms, or ventricular septal defect (VSD). The nurse may be the first to recognize a systolic murmur in combination with a deteriorating condition post myocardial infarction. These signs may be indicative of a VSD or mitral regurgitation that could be managed with an IABP pending surgery. The nurse may suggest that an IABP be considered for the patient who continues to demonstrate an increased pulmonary capillary wedge pressure and decreased cardiac output. She/he may also suggest the use of an IABP for a patient with unstable angina awaiting coronary bypass grafting or the high risk patient undergoing cardiac diagnostic studies.

In addition, the initial management of post cardiac surgery patients sometimes includes use of the intra-aortic balloon pump to increase cardiac output. The IABP may also be used to augment cardiac function prophylactically during non-cardiac surgery and in high risk patients undergoing cardiac catheterization or coronary angioplasty.(9–12)

Contraindications to the IABP include aortic insufficiency, thoracic or abdominal aortic dissection, or aortic aneurysm. With aortic valve incompetence, blood enters the left ventricle during diastole, and with

Table 7.1

Indications for Counterpulsation
Intractable unstable angina
Intractable ventricular arrhythmias
Pump failure due to:
complications of myocardial infarction
viral myocarditis
idiopathic myocarditis
low cardiac output syndrome
end-stage cardiomyopathy
Acute mechanical defects
chordeal rupture
mitral regurgitation
ventricular septal rupture
Perioperative support and stabilization
cardiac catheterization
coronary angioplasty
cardiac surgery
general surgery in high-risk cardiac patients
bridge to cardiac transplantation

diastolic augmentation the regurgitant volume increases. In the presence of an aortic aneurysm or dissection, counterpulsation may cause expansion of the aneurysm or rupture. Some consider the presence of a prosthetic aortic valve a contraindication for an IABP (13); however, this view is not universal. Severe peripheral vascular disease is a relative contraindication for an IABP due to the increased potential for vascular and aortic damage. Certain arrhythmias, including atrial fibrillation, atrial tachycardia, and chaotic rhythms present a relative contraindication, as the rhythm disturbance must be controlled for optimal functioning of the IABP. It is also difficult to achieve satisfactory pumping with brady-arrhythmias less than 60 or heart rates greater than 110. It is the role of the critical care nurse to alert the attending physician or cardiologist to any of these conditions, and to be aware of the increased risks related to the use of the IABP in these patients (Table 7.2).

Balloon Description

Intra-aortic balloon catheters are constructed of a siliconized polyurethane material that minimizes the danger of clot formation on the balloon surface. Multiple size options are available, with a balloon volume of 20 to 50 cc, membrane length of 9 to 10.3 inches (228–260 mm), and inflated diameters of 15 to 18 mm. The balloons are mounted on No. 8, 9, 10, and 12 French catheters, with smaller sizes available for pediatric

Table 7.2

Contraindications for Counterpulsation

Definite:
  Aortic insufficiency
  Aortic dissection
  Aortic aneurysm

Relative
  Prosthetic aortic valve

With caution in
  Peripheral vascular disease
  Certain arrhythmias
  Bleeding disorders
  Thrombocytopenia

Table 7.3

Determination of Balloon Size

Age × Weight (lb)	Balloon Size (cc)
<3500	20
3500–6000	30
>6000	40

use. The balloon size is selected according to total body surface area and the size of the femoral artery upon exploration (Table 7.3). An echocardiogram may be useful to evaluate aortic dimensions before selection of balloon size.

Double lumen catheters enhance patient safety during insertion and throughout the course of IABP therapy. The two lumens permit visualization of the arterial pressure during insertion with simultaneous use of a guide wire via the central lumen. Central aortic timing is possible, which eliminates the need for peripheral arterial monitoring.

Patient Preparation and Insertion Procedure

Percutaneous insertion of the intra-aortic balloon catheter has been demonstrated to be highly successful and it allows rapid initiation of counterpulsation. The inflatable balloon is inserted into the descending thoracic aorta, with the tip placement just distal to the left subclavian artery. The catheter may also be inserted at the bedside by surgical cut-down technique. This method is sometimes preferable if the patient has severe peripheral atherosclerosis. In this approach, the physician performs a femoral arteriotomy through which to pass the catheter. A dacron graft may be inserted in the arteriotomy site to prevent vessel collapse.

In most instances, the invasive cardiologist or cardiovascular surgeon will insert the balloon catheter. A cardiology fellow, resident physician, or surgical nurse will act as the second assistant. The critical care nurse functions as the balloon nurse. She/he performs the start-up procedure and continues patient care throughout the insertion, including monitoring and administration of medication. Nursing measures during the insertion and post-insertion are the same for either the percutaneous or cutdown approach.

Before insertion, the nurse ascertains the patency and accessibility of intravenous (IV) lines for emergency medications if needed during the procedure. It is important to keep drapes away from the injection ports and maintain clear access to the peripheral IV. If the patient is on a ventilator, the nurse checks the settings and alarms, drains the tubing, and suctions the patient before the insertion. A baseline pulse oximetry reading or arterial blood gas will be useful for later assessment of balloon effectiveness.

The patient's groin is prepped before draping. Excess hair may be clipped or shaved, and the area cleansed with a povidone-iodine solution. A local anesthetic is then administered, as well as IV sedation if indicated. The balloon integrity is tested before insertion by inflating it with the desired amount of air and checking for leaks. This is done under aseptic conditions by the physician.

Complications during Insertion

Complications may occur during insertion, including an inability to insert the catheter, resulting in emboli, aortoiliac dissection, circulatory obstruction, arterial perforation, and balloon malposition (Table 7.4).(14) Patients must be carefully assessed for signs and symptoms of these situations, including chest pain or back pain. A chest radiograph, fluoroscopy, or transesophageal echocardiography is done immediately after insertion to verify balloon position.(7, 15)

The patient's cardiac rhythm, blood pressure, and clinical status are monitored throughout the procedure for early recognition and management of complications. The physician is promptly alerted to any significant change in status or pain. For example, acute back pain, flank pain, or testicular pain (in men) may signify aortic dissection, warranting immediate notification of the physician. Vasovagal responses secondary to aortic stimulation during the catheter passage may require atropine.

Table 7.4

Complications of the Intra-aortic Balloon Pump
Aortic dissection or rupture
Emboli
Vascular obstruction
Bleeding
Thrombocytopenia
Local infection
Systemic infection

Console and Transducer Preparation

The IABP console is prepared for start-up by establishing the power and selecting the electrocardiogram (ECG) trigger, unless the physician indicates otherwise. The trigger is the physiologically related signal that serves to activate balloon inflation and deflation. The console will provide a message or audible sound that the self test has been completed. The helium tank is opened and the initial control settings established.

The arterial transducer for the central aortic arterial line is assembled and then attached via the interface to the IABP console. Electrocardiogram input to the IABP console is established directly, via the patient cable. The patient electrodes are positioned to obtain the ECG configuration with the maximal R wave amplitude and minimal amplitude of all other waves and artifact. The positive deflection of the R wave triggers balloon deflation, regardless of the patient's rhythm. Two sources of ECG are needed—one on the bedside monitor and one on the console.

Flush System and Attachments

The double lumen balloon catheter consists of an outside lumen for driving gas delivery and a central aortic lumen for pressure monitoring that is situated inside the gas channel. After the catheter has been inserted, a continuous flush system is attached to the central aortic lumen stopcock, per the following procedure.

The central aortic lumen stopcock is turned to the "off" position to the aortic lumen during the connection. A 10-cc syringe filled with flush solution is attached to the side port of the central aortic lumen stopcock. The aortic lumen is then aspirated to ensure patency and eliminate air trapped in the stopcock. Smaller syringes are to be avoided, as they may produce higher pressures during flushing. If the nurse is unable to aspirate the lumen, the physician is notified and the lumen stopcock turned off. If the lumen is easily aspirated, the flush by syringe is completed, then the aortic lumen stopcock is "opened" to the flush system. The side port of the lumen stopcock is capped with a sterile Luer-Lock cap. The flush system must remain air free at all times.

The IABP catheter is attached with an extender through the flex relief bracket to the safety chamber of the IABP console. No other adaptors are placed on the line as extensions increase dead space and therefore increase inflation time. The driving gas lines are evacuated and purged according to the console manufacturer's instructions.

Pumping is initiated at low volume (10 cc) of driving gas, and gradually increased until the desired amount (20 to 50 cc) is achieved. Low volume minimizes potential trauma to the aorta. The nurse must observe closely for blood in the gas delivery catheter, as this line is connected to the balloon itself and the presence of blood is highly indicative of a balloon leak.

Blood in the central aortic arterial catheter is not unexpected, and may be cleared by flushing the system and assuring that all connections are secure. However, inadvertent disconnections may result in serious blood loss. Continuous pressure monitoring with alarms is mandatory throughout the course of the IABP therapy for detection of accidental disconnection.

Post Insertion Management
After the IABP counterpulsation has been initiated, the peripheral pulses are assessed, compared with the pre-IABP status, and the quality documented. A sterile dressing is applied to the groin site according to hospital policy and procedure for central lines. Intra-aortic balloon catheters must be taped securely to the leg and further stabilized by a leg splint to prevent displacement.

Patient and Family Teaching
Patient teaching subsequent to the balloon insertion will primarily relate to forced immobility. The patient can be instructed that he/she may move in the bed, but bed rest must be maintained and the hip on the affected side can not be flexed more than 30 degrees. He will be unable to bend his legs or sit up. The patient is encouraged to move within his limits, however, as some patients will be reluctant to move at all without reassurance from the nurse.

The patient and his family members will also benefit from a simple explanation at this point of the balloon function and console operation. It is helpful to familiarize them with the normal operating sounds of the console and describe the alarm functions.

Psychological Support
The patient who is treated with an intra-aortic balloon pump may have anxieties about both his medical condition and his treatment. He will

have questions regarding his survival and morbidity, and may be antici-
pating surgery or percutaneous coronary angioplasty. He may be dis-
turbed by the thought of having a foreign device in his aorta. He may be
concerned about his family members, his financial liabilities, or his job.

It is important that the nurse provide a calm, restful environment for the
patient. She/he can provide planned periods of uninterrupted rest, and
reassure the patient simply by her knowledgeable presence. Both the
patient and his family members will appreciate frequent communication
from the staff members, and explanations of all that is occurring. The
nurse remains alert to the patient's specific questions, and provides thorough answers herself or relays the questions to the appropriate health
care professional. It is also helpful to share positive information with the
patient and his family members, such as improvements in his angina,
skin color, or urine output. Some patients find liberalized visiting hours
to be of comfort.

Patient Maintenance during IABP Therapy

The longer the time a patient is maintained on the IABP, the greater is
the risk of complications. These include vascular complications, fatal aortic perforations, leg ischemia, bleeding from the femoral artery,
hematomas, and infection or septicemia.(2, 16, 17) Nursing responsibilities during this phase of therapy include frequent head to toe assess-
ments, maintenance of devices, and the provision of routine patient care.
Several broad categories of special concern are described in the following text.

Achievement of Hemodynamic Stability

The nurse evaluates and documents clinical and hemodynamic responses to IABP therapy every 15 to 60 minutes and as indicated. Monitoring
parameters include routine vital signs, central venous pressure, pulmonary artery pressure, pulmonary capillary wedge pressure (PCWP),
thermodilution cardiac output, mixed venous oxygen saturation, body
temperature, intake and output, and laboratory values. The cuff blood
pressure should be compared with the console pressure every 4 hours.

Physiological parameters may improve within 15 minutes of initiation of
IABP therapy. Clinical signs and symptoms of improvement include a
heart rate less than 110 per minute, a cardiac index greater than 2.0
$L/min/m^2$, ventricular ectopy less than 6 beats per minute, improvement
in oxygenation, and a decreased PCWP. The patient may also demonstrate relief from angina, and require little or no inotropic support.(6)

The patient is monitored for cardiac arrhythmias, as the potential for cardiac arrest exists. If cardiac arrest does occur, cardiopulmonary resuscitation is initiated and the internal console trigger used for inflation and

deflation of the balloon. This will also minimize clot formation that would otherwise occur with a dormant balloon catheter. Vasopressors may be administered as ordered and titrated according to mean arterial pressure.

Maintenance of Renal Function

An improvement in renal function may be noted after initiation of IABP therapy, reflective of an improved cardiac output. However, use of the intra-aortic balloon catheter may also result in renal dysfunction, due to renal thromboemboli or slippage of the balloon catheter and obstruction of the renal arteries. Occult blood by urinalysis or an elevated blood urea nitrogen and creatinine, and active bleeding or an anemia evident by laboratory result are promptly reported.

Prevention of Vascular Complications

The most common complications of IABP therapy are vascular in nature, including extension or rupture of an aortic aneurysm, rupture or perforation of the femoral or iliac arteries, gas embolism resulting from IAB rupture, and occlusion of the femoral artery.(3) Aortic dissection or perforation may be manifested by sudden and severe abdominal pain or back pain, hypotension, tachycardia, and a falling hematocrit.(18)

Nursing measures to reduce balloon tears will also reduce the incidence of gas emboli. The physician must be given adequate assistance during the balloon insertion, and the balloon should remain out of the operative field during the procedure to prevent accidental tearing by the instruments. Nursing assessment post-procedure includes monitoring for signs and symptoms of distal, peripheral emboli. The external balloon of the console is checked every 2 hours for a smooth, taut appearance, which indicates an intact internal balloon.

Small balloon leaks may be detected post-insertion by the appearance of blood in the gas delivery catheter. If this occurs, pumping is stopped immediately, the physician notified, and the patient placed in Trendelenburg's position until the balloon is removed.(14) In this position, the driving gas (helium or carbon dioxide) is displaced from the central circulation toward the periphery.

The critical care nurse is responsible for frequent assessment of the pulses, color, sensation, movement, capillary filling time, and temperature of the affected limb. Claudication should be noted. Her early observations may be instrumental in the prevention of arterial injury, limb ischemia, and hematomas.

Lower limb ischemia is a frequent complication of IABP therapy and detrimental consequences can persist long after hospitalization. (19) One case of acute lower body ischemia has been reported, due to persistent balloon inflation throughout the cardiac cycle, resulting in distal aortic occlusion.(20)

The quality of posterior tibial and dorsalis pedis pulses in both extremities is assessed every 15 minutes for the first hour after insertion, every 30 minutes for 2 hours, and then every hour while the intra-aortic balloon catheter is in place. Doppler flow technique may be necessary to detect weak pulses. Loss of perfusion to the extremity may necessitate balloon catheter removal. New advances in intra-aortic balloon catheter design, including smaller catheters and sheathless insertion, may reduce the incidence of limb ischemia.(7) The soft tissue of the cannulated extremity can also be protected by means of a sheepskin pad or foot cradle.

Prevention of Bleeding, Hematomas, and Thrombocytopenia

A pressure dressing is applied to the balloon insertion site immediately post-procedure, and replaced every 24 hours or as necessary. Bleeding precautions are initiated due to the anticoagulant therapy. Frank bleeding is noted and reported promptly.

Clotting studies are periodically drawn (every 6 hours while the heparin dose is adjusted then every 12 to 24 hours while the IABP remains in place), with the target partial thromboplastin time usually desirable at 1 1/2 to 2 times the control. The platelet count is also closely monitored, with a desirable level over 150,000 per mL. A hemoglobin and hematocrit should be drawn at least daily.

If hemorrhage occurs, blood products are administered as ordered. Platelet counts usually return to baseline soon after the IABP therapy is discontinued.(14)

Maintenance of Adequate Oxygenation

The critical care nurse monitors for signs of respiratory insufficiency. The lung sounds are auscultated every 4 hours and as needed. Rales and rhonchi may be indicative of pulmonary congestion due to progressive myocardial failure.(18) The arterial blood gas is monitored and oxygen administered as ordered. Routine respiratory care is performed with minor modifications of position. The head of the bed should not be elevated more than 15 degrees nor should the involved leg be flexed.

Often times the IABP patient is also intubated and ventilated.

Respiratory failure in the IABP patient is most commonly of cardiac origin, and the respiratory status is expected to improve as hemodynamic stability is obtained. The critical care nurse will manage the ventilator as she/he would for any patient with acute respiratory distress.

Prevention of Infection

Careful handwashing before patient contact is essential. Any dressing changes are carried out with aseptic technique. Universal precautions are maintained, with the use of gloves, gowns, and masks when indicated to prevent the transmission of blood-borne pathogens, such as hepatitis B and human immunodeficiency virus. Antibiotics are administered as ordered, including prophylactic use. Careful attention to patient hygiene will include aseptic Foley catheter care and peripheral IV line and dressing changes. The patient's temperature is closely monitored, as well as the white blood cell count, for elevation. The intra-aortic balloon catheter insertion site is covered with a sterile occlusive dressing and changed daily. Local tenderness, swelling, or purulent drainage may suggest infection.

Blood specimens are withdrawn from a peripheral arterial line or venipuncture whenever possible. The central aortic catheter lumen may be used for this purpose only if ordered by the physician. Aseptic technique must be adhered to when blood specimens are withdrawn from the intra-aortic balloon line. After withdrawal, the aspiration port is flushed, as blood remaining in the port is an ideal medium for bacterial growth. All ports of all stopcocks are covered with sterile caps at all times.

Prevention of Problems Related to Immobility and Maintenance of Catheter Integrity

In order to prevent displacement of the intra-aortic balloon catheter, the nurse assures that the head of the patient's bed is raised no more than 30 degrees, that the patient turn toward the insertion side only, and that there be no flexing of the hip. There should be some slack in the catheter, and positioning the console at the foot of the bed is usually very effective for maximizing access to the patient. If a disconnection occurs, the catheter is reconnected immediately and the system purged to refill the balloon, before pumping is resumed.

Damage to the aortic arch may occur related to the stiffness of the balloon catheter and its sharp tip, particularly in patients with atherosclerosis. Catheters may also crack with flexion, resulting in gas leakage and ineffective pumping.(3) To help minimize these complications, the patient's leg may be loosely restrained below the insertion site. The patient is logrolled, and the affected leg supported while turning, maintaining good alignment. If blood appears in the connecting tubing at any time, pumping is discontinued and the physician notified immediately.

To reduce the effects of immobility, the patient is generally turned every hour, and range of motion is provided to all extremities every 4 hours. An egg crate mattress or air mattress may be considered. The patient is instructed and encouraged in the use of cough and deep breathing exercises or incentive spirometry every 2 hours. Very restless patients may require sedatives for their anxiety.

Maintenance of Level of Consciousness

The nurse's role in the care of the IABP patient includes prevention of the disorientation that may occur in any critical care unit patient.

Table 7.5

Determinants of Effective Pumping
Volume of driving gas
Elasticity of aortic wall
Left ventricular stroke volume
Intra-aortic blood pressure
Systemic vascular resistance
Heart rate and rhythm
Balloon location
Balloon length and size

Neurological status is assessed at least once every 8 hours. Simple reorientation techniques, such as talking with the patient, placing a clock and calendar within eyesight, and providing a television, radio, and newspapers are in order. Prompt recognition and treatment of delirium is essential.

At least one third of patients receiving IABP counterpulsation have been shown to demonstrate delirium severe enough to require treatment.(21) The etiology of this delirium is unclear, but possible causes include altered cerebral blood flow related to a change in cardiac output or the counterpulsation itself, the release of humoral factors due to the foreign body in the aorta, and the restlessness that may accompany forced bed rest. The delirium usually occurs within the first two days of IABP therapy, and is unrelated to the age of the patient. Untreated delirium may lead to further cardiovascular compromise and the patient may endanger his own safety. The current treatment of choice is rapid tranquilization with intravenous haloperidol. Family members should be reassured that the delirium usually clears shortly after the IABP therapy is discontinued.(21, 22)

Maintenance of Optimal Balloon Pumping
The effectiveness of balloon pumping is determined by both patient hemodynamics and equipment issues (Table 7.5). Augmentation limits are selected on the console and alarms are left on at all times. Intra-aortic balloon pump timing is evaluated hourly, and adjusted as needed, by balloon certified personnel only, from the central aortic lumen pressure waveform.

Balloon inactivity is limited to a period less than 15 minutes. In the event of console malfunction or loss of electricity, the nurse must manually inflate then deflate the balloon with a 60-cc syringe. Using a three-way stopcock and 40 cc of air, the balloon is inflated then deflated once every 5 minutes.

Newer model balloon consoles may be set to an automatic timing mode. Although this eases the constant surveillance necessary with manual timing, the critical care nurse must still ensure that this timing is optimal, so that the patient receives the maximum benefit from the IABP. The waveform is assessed frequently.

In order to evaluate IABP timing, it is necessary to first understand the normal arterial waveform and the significance of its components, which are illustrated in Figure 7.1. The tracing begins with the systolic upstroke and peak systolic pressure, which correlate with left ventricular contraction and ejection. This is followed by systolic runoff, when systolic ejection continues at a reduced pressure and volume. The dicrotic notch represents aortic valve closure, with the end of systole and onset of diastole. Ventricular relaxation and filling occur during the diastolic phase.(23)

Intra-aortic balloon pump timing refers to adjustments that are made to synchronize the inflate/deflate cycle of the IABP with the patient's own hemodynamics. It is adjusted while using the central aortic waveform. Aortic pressure reflects real time in the cardiac cycle, whereas radial arterial pressure on the bedside monitor is delayed.

Balloon timing is best assessed with a 1:2 augmented mode, as per Figure 7.2. With this setting, the first waveform (a) will represent the patient's own unassisted pressures. The following waveform (b) will demonstrate balloon assisted pressures. With proper timing, the augmented wave or balloon inflation will begin at the dicrotic notch. The augmented pressure

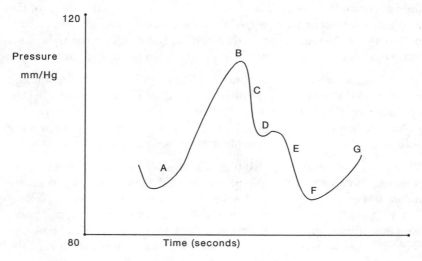

Figure 7.1. *Normal arterial waveform.*

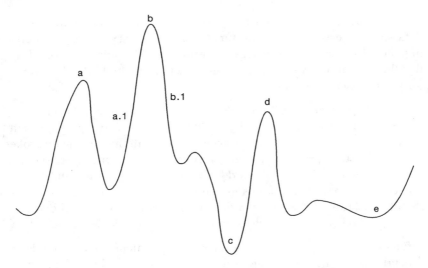

Figure 7.2. *Balloon timing strip with 1:2 augmentation.*

tracing will show an increase in aortic pressure, which raises coronary artery perfusion. Balloon deflation will create a reduction in aortic end-diastolic pressure (c), or afterload reduction, and a subsequent reduction in the peak pressure of the following systole (d), or systolic unloading. The augmented wave should result in a 5- to 10-mm drop, or presystolic dip, in the aortic end-diastolic pressure.(18, 24) With proper timing, the assist-ed systolic pressure will be less than the unassisted patient systolic pres-sure, and the balloon assisted aortic end-diastolic pressure will be less than the patient aortic end-diastolic pressure (e). The beneficial effects of the augmentation will be an increased diastolic pressure, stroke volume, coro-nary perfusion pressure, and cardiac output. There will also be reductions in myocardial oxygen consumption (MVO_2), afterload, and preload.

The calibration and timing of balloon inflation and deflation is monitored and recorded at least every 4 hours. It should also be reassessed whenev-er there are changes in the patient's hemodynamic profile or cardiac rhythm. If inappropriate timing is found, inflation and deflation times are readjusted and the physician notified of any serious complications.

With late inflation of the IABP (Fig. 7.3), the period of diastolic augmen-tation is shortened, with subsequent reduced therapeutic effects. Early inflation (Fig. 7.4), before the closure of the aortic valve, is more deleteri-ous, with increased myocardial stress, decreased cardiac output, and possi-ble intracardiac shunting if mechanical defects are present. Early deflation (Fig. 7.5), before isovolumetric contraction, will reduce the therapeutic effects of counterpulsation. With late deflation (Fig. 7.6), ejection is

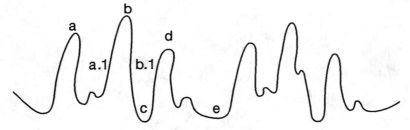

Figure 7.3. *Late inflation.*

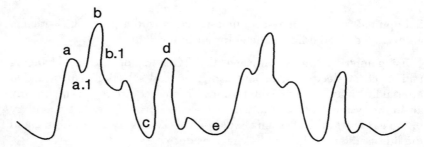

Figure 7.4. *Early inflation.*

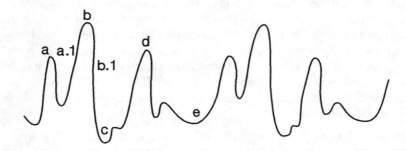

Figure 7.5. *Early deflation.*

impeded, MVO_2 is increased, and there may be adverse hemodynamic consequences in patients who have true ventricular aneurysm, mitral regurgitation, or ventricular septal defect.

Reduced augmentation may also occur in the presence of optimal timing. The waveform will fail to demonstrate a reduced assisted end-diastolic pressure or patient systolic pressure. Possible causes include incorrect balloon size or placement, a reduced balloon volume, hypertension, or hypovolemia.

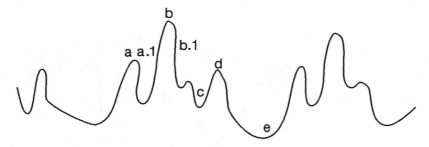

Figure 7.6. *Late deflation.*

Suboptimal pumping may also be associated with a poor ECG tracing, an occluded arterial line catheter, or air in the system.

Nursing interventions to improve the ECG tracing include changing patient chest electrodes, patient cable, or lead selection. An occluded arterial line may improve with flushing or may require replacement. Any air in the system must be purged as described previously. The adequacy of the gas level in the system should be checked every 2 to 4 hours, and the lines refilled or the tank changed as necessary.

Balloon timing and pumping are best achieved with a patient in normal sinus rhythm at a rate of 90 to 110. Equally beneficial results can be obtained with an atrial or atrioventricular sequential paced rhythm through the use of the pacer rejection trigger mode. However, when the heart rate exceeds 120 per minute for carbon dioxide systems, or 140 per minute for helium systems, there is decreased gas volume and therefore decreased balloon volume. In these situations, augmentation may be increased by decreasing the balloon assist rate from 1:1 to 1:2. Some console models are designed to overcome this difficulty by the delivery of higher gas shuttle speeds.

The most difficult rhythm for balloon pumping is an atrial fibrillation at a rate of 80 to 120. To address this issue, signal detection can be inhibited for a set interval following trigger generation, so that balloon inflation occurs at a specific time after the previous deflation. If the atrial fibrillation rate approaches 120 to 140, it may be helpful to change the assist rate to 1:2.

Maintain Devices
The nurse's responsibilities may extend beyond the patient himself to care of the console, pulmonary artery catheter, peripheral arterial line, and gas tank. Evaluation of the pumping capability of the console and trouble-shooting may be necessary. Problems that are strictly related to the equipment and appropriate nursing interventions are summarized in Table 7.6. (7, 8, 25)

Table 7.6

Troubleshooting for the Intra-aortic Balloon Pump

Equipment Problem	Possible Causes: Non-Patient Related	Nursing Intervention
Decreased augmentation	Overdamping	(1) Check tubing for blood, kinking, or condensation. (2) Check for air bubble, cracks, or leaks in system, including transducer. (3) Tighten all connections. (4) Fast flush lines. (5) Recalibrate transducer q 4 h.
	Balloon volume	(1) Check balloon volume every 2 h and refill as necessary.
Premature balloon deflation	Atrial pacer spikes sensed as R waves	(1) Choose lead with spike in opposite direction (usually Lead II), or switch to arterial pressure trigger.
Inaccurate monitor pressures	Underdamping	(1) Recalibrate transducer.
Mechanical IABP console malfunction	Equipment failure	(1) Manually inflate and deflate balloon with syringe until console can be replaced. (2) Contact manufacturer.
Appearance of blood in catheter	Balloon rupture	(1) Stop pumping. (2) Clamp catheter. (3) Notify physician immediately. (4) Prepare to remove balloon.
Loss of cardiac signal	Loose lead	(1) Check patient leads and replace as necessary.

Documentation

Descriptive documentation is made at a frequency of at least every 4 hours. This includes lung sounds, skin color and temperature, mentation, appearance of insertion site and cannulated extremity, peripheral pulses and pain. An accurate intake and output are charted at 1-hour intervals. The vital signs are recorded at least hourly along with the balloon ratio setting.

The systolic, diastolic and mean pressure numbers are recorded from the IABP console. Appropriate timing is documented with a timing strip mounted in the progress notes every 4 hours and whenever the ratio is adjusted. The strip is labelled with the patient's name, date, time, and scale (40 or 80 mm Hg per centimeter). The waveform on the timing strip can be labelled as follows for one assisted cardiac cycle:

1 = unassisted patient systolic pressure,
2 = peak diastolic augmented pressure,
3 = balloon assisted aortic end-diastolic pressure,
4 = assisted systolic pressure, and
5 = patient aortic end-diastolic pressure.

Patient Transport

Patients may require in-hospital transport to other departments, such as nuclear medicine or the cardiac catheterization laboratory. They may also be transported to other institutions for surgery or testing. In either scenario, the patient who is receiving IABP therapy should always travel in the escort of at least one critical care nurse, and preferably a physician. Many ambulance companies have mobile intensive care unit vans that are equipped with IABPs and advanced cardiac life support (ACLS) equipment for interagency transport. However, in the absence of these necessities, the hospital IABP console will usually function on battery or auxiliary power for 45 to 60 minutes. The personnel traveling with the patient must be prepared to trouble-shoot the balloon, manually inflate and deflate the balloon if necessary, and administer lifesaving medications, cardiopulmonary resuscitation, and defibrillation.

Weaning

Predictors of successful weaning from the IABP are a PCWP less than 18 mm Hg, cardiac index greater than 2.2, and systolic blood pressure (BP) greater than 90.(26) The weaning protocol will be ordered by the physician. A standard routine is to systematically reduce the ratio of assisted heart beats to the total number of heart beats from 1:1 to 1:2 and eventually 1:4. This is called frequency ratio weaning, and is sometimes recommended to decrease the incidence of clot formation around the balloon.(13) Weaning may be completed in as little as 60 minutes. If the weaning time is prolonged, the mode should be returned to 1:1 for 5 minutes each hour to reduce the incidence of clot formation. If the patient demonstrates hemodynamic independence on the 1:4 mode, removal of the IABP is indicated.

Another weaning method is to gradually reduce the augmentation volume rather than the ratio. This method is viewed by some practitioners as more physiologic as the heart gradually resumes its circulatory load.(13) Care must be taken not to decrease the volume to the point of balloon stasis. The nurse periodically observes the safety chamber of the console for fluctuation of the external balloon.

Patients who are being treated with IABP therapy are frequently managed with vasoactive and inotropic drugs, in addition to ventilatory support. It is recommended that these supports be weaned one at a time, rather than in combination with weaning from the IABP.(26) It is also common for chemical afterload reduction to be initiated or increased concurrently with the IABP weaning. For example, the nurse may be titrating IV nitroprusside or administering angiotensin converting enzyme inhibitors at the same time that IABP weaning is in progress.

Intolerance of weaning may be manifested by a decreasing BP, increased heart rate, increased PCWP, decreased cardiac output, decreased oxygen level, decreased urine output, clouding of the sensorium, angina, ST segment or T wave changes, cold clammy skin of the extremities, and new onset of dysrhythmias. The nursing action if these symptoms appear is to return the timing to 1:1 or the augmentation volume to its original setting and notify the physician.(6)

Removal of IABP Therapy

While awaiting balloon removal, it is recommended that a minimal inflation rate of 1:4 or 1:8 be maintained to prevent clotting. Before removing the balloon, the patient's clotting profile is evaluated and any abnormalities corrected. This will minimize the risk of bleeding. Anticoagulant therapy is tapered, and heparin drips are usually discontinued approximately 4 hours before removal of the intra-aortic balloon catheter.

After organizing the equipment, the nurse will turn the IABP console off when ordered, and aspirate the balloon using a one-way valve or three-way stopcock with a 60-cc syringe to create a vacuum. The sutures will be removed at the insertion site, and the balloon and the sheath will be withdrawn as a unit by the physician under aseptic conditions. The site is allowed to bleed for 3 seconds before pressure is applied, to permit removal of any clot. Direct manual compression of the femoral artery is then applied for 30 minutes, or longer if bleeding persists. The puncture site is not checked at shorter intervals to see if bleeding reoccurs, because hematoma formation makes further arterial compression more difficult and less efficient. After 15 minutes of compression, however, pressure is briefly eased in order to allow perfusion of the lower extremity.

The nurse evaluates the peripheral pulses and patient status immediately after the IABP removal. The physician is notified immediately for the loss of pulses or patient deterioration. After apparent cessation of bleeding, the puncture site remains under direct visualization for another 10 minutes. An expanding hematoma implies bleeding and direct compression is required for an additional 20 minutes.

When hemostasis is assured, a sterile pressure dressing is applied to the groin site and a 5-pound sandbag placed over the dressing for 6 hours. The insertion site is assessed for bleeding every 30 minutes times 2, then hourly times 8, then every 4 hours times 6. Again, if there is any evidence of bleeding, compression is applied to the site and the physician notified. The head of the bed must remain less than 30 degrees elevated and the affected leg is not flexed for 18 additional hours. Bed rest is recommended for this period. The nurse continues to monitor for bleeding, occlusion, or infection at the site for a period of 48 hours.

New Advances in Counterpulsation

The automatic timing mechanisms of the new balloon pump consoles have significantly decreased the nursing time necessary for management of equipment. Most models will automatically inflate and deflate at the appropriate times unless the automatic timing mechanism is manually overridden. They adjust for delays if the trigger is slaved off a bedside monitor, and adjust for changes in heart rate and rhythm. Some automatically check the balloon gas level and purge and fill the system at 2-hour intervals.(8)

These technological advances may result in less nursing care hours required per patient. However, it is still essential that all nurses caring for patients on IABPs have completed a course in the principles of counterpulsation. The possibility of equipment failure will always exist, and staff must be prepared to deal with such emergencies.

Intra-aortic Balloon Pump Certification Process

All hospital personnel involved with setting, adjusting the timing of the IABP, and trouble-shooting problems with the pumps should be IABP certified by the individual hospital. Before beginning the certification process, it is recommended that the nurse have at least 6 months experience on a critical care unit and have successfully completed an ACLS course.

The certification process itself will include self-directed study through completion of assigned readings, and attendance at a formal IABP course. This is followed by supervised experiences caring for a patient with an IABP, under the direction of a balloon certified nurse. A performance checklist is completed, and the nurse will be able to obtain timing strips and chart appropriate information.

Nursing Diagnoses

A list of potential nursing diagnoses for the patient on an IABP is presented in the following text. Appropriate patient-specific goals and nursing interventions can be developed by following the usual nursing process.

1. Decreased cardiac output related to decreased myocardial contractility, dysrhythmias, and/or ineffective IABP timing.
2. Alteration in tissue perfusion (cardiopulmonary, renal, peripheral, and/or cerebral) related to decreased blood flow secondary to catheter position.
3. High risk for impaired skin integrity related to immobility.
4. High risk for injury related to potential retroperitoneal bleed or bleeding from femoral balloon insertion site exacerbated by anticoagulant therapy.
5. Altered pattern of urinary elimination related to Foley catheter.
6. Bathing/hygiene self care deficit related to activity restrictions.
7. Sleep pattern disturbance related to alarms, activity restrictions, and discomfort.
8. High risk for infection related to invasive lines.
9. Anxiety related to disease process and perceived health status.
10. Knowledge deficit related to therapeutic interventions.

(8, 27)

Summary

In summary, care of the IABP patient can be both professionally stimulating and rewarding. It provides the nursing staff with the opportunity to exercise and improve their knowledge and skills in physical assessment, patient teaching and support, and the coordination and monitoring of multiple invasive devices. The focus of this chapter has been on those aspects of the care of the IABP patient that are almost exclusively nursing in nature. The reader is referred to the other chapters of this book for greater detail on the multidisciplinary areas of patient management.

REFERENCES

1. Braunwald E. Heart Disease. 2nd ed. Philadelphia: WB Saunders; 1984.
2. Eltchaninoff H, Dimas AP, Whitlow PL. Complications associated with percutaneous placement and use of intraaortic balloon counterpulsation. Am J Cardiol 1993;71(4):328–332.
3. Haak SW. Intra-aortic balloon pump techniques. Dimensions Crit Care Nurs 1983;2(4):196–204.
4. Kahn JK, Rutherford BD, McConahay DR, Johnson WL, Giorgi LV, Hartzler GO. Supported "high risk" coronary angioplasty using intraaortic balloon pump counterpulsation. J Am Coll Cardiol 1990; 15(5):1151–1155.
5. Mueller HS. Role of intra-aortic counterpulsation in cardiogenic shock and acute myocardial infarction. Cardiology 1994;84(3):168–174.
6. Schott KE. Intra-aortic balloon counterpulsation as a therapy for shock. Crit Care Nurs Clin North Am 1990;2(2):187–193.

7. Shinn AE, Joseph D. Concepts of intraaortic balloon counterpulsation. J Cardiovasc Nurs 1994;8(2):45–60.

8. Shoulders-Odom B. Managing the challenge of IABP therapy. Crit Care Nurse 1991;11(2):50–52, 64–76.

9. Aguirre FV, Kern MJ, Bach R, et al. Intraaortic balloon pump support during high-risk coronary angioplasty. Cardiology 1994; 84(3):175–186.

10. Georgeson S, Coombs AT, Eckman MH. Prophylactic use of the intra-aortic balloon pump in high-risk cardiac patients undergoing noncardiac surgery: A decision analytic view. Am J Med 1992;92(6): 665–678.

11. Ohman EM, George BS, White CJ, et al. Use of aortic counterpulsation to improve sustained coronary artery patency during acute myocardial infarction. Results of a randomized trial. The Randomized IABP Study Group. Circulation 1994;90(2):792–799.

12. Underwood MJ, Firmin RK, Graham TR. Current concepts in the use of intra-aortic balloon counterpulsation. Br J Hosp Med 1993; 50(7):391–397.

13. Kantrowitz A, Cardonna RR, Freed PS. Percutaneous intra-aortic balloon counterpulsation. Crit Care Clin 1992;8(4):819–837.

14. Bullas JB. Care of the patient on the percutaneous intra-aortic counterpulsation balloon. Crit Care Nurse 1982;2(4):40-48.

15. Shanewise JS, Sadel SM. Intraoperative transesophageal echocardiography to assist the insertion and positioning of the intraaortic balloon pump. Anesth Analg 1994;79(3):577–580.

16. Aksnes J, Abdelnoor M, Berge V, Fjeld NB. Risk factors of septicemia and perioperative myocardial infarction in a cohort of patients supported with intra-aortic balloon (IABP) in the course of open heart surgery. Eur J Cardiothorac Surg 1993;7(3):153–157.

17. Barnett MG, Swartz MT, Peterson GJ, et al. Vascular complications from intraaortic balloons: Risk analysis. J Vasc Surg 1994;19(1):81–89.

18. Thompson JM, McFarland GK, Hirsh JE, Tucker SM. Mosby's Clinical Nursing. 3rd ed. St. Louis: Mosby-Year Book; 1993.

19. Funk M, Ford CF, Foell DW, et al. Frequency of long-term lower limb ischemia associated with intraaortic balloon pump use. Am J Cardiol 1992;70(13):1195–1199.

20. Ferrell MA, Doherty M, Zusman RM, Nash IS. Total aortic occlusion caused by sustained balloon inflation: A previously unreported complication of intraaortic balloon counterpulsation. Cathet Cardiovasc Diagn 1993;30(3): 211–213.

21. Sanders KM, Stern TA, O'Gara PT, et al. Delirium during intra-aortic balloon pump therapy. Psychosomatics 1992;33(1):35–44.

22. Sanders KM, Stern TA. Management of delirium associated with use of the intra-aortic balloon pump. Am J Crit Care 1993;2(5):371 –377.

23. Wojner AW. Assessing the five points of the intra-aortic balloon pump waveform. Crit Care Nurse 1994;14(3):48–52.

24. Thomas S. Intra-aortic balloon pumps. Nurs Standard 1993; 8(8):50–51.

25. Joseph DL, Bates S. Intra aortic balloon pumping. How to stay on course. Am J Nurs 1990;90(9):42–47.

26. Bavin TK, Self MA. Weaning from intra-aortic balloon pump support. Am J Nurs 1991;91(10):54–59.

27. Potter PA, Perry AG. Fundamentals of Nursing. Concepts, Process & Practice. 3rd ed. St. Louis: Mosby Year Book; 1993.

8

Ventricular Assist Devices

David M. Fehr ▪ Kane M. High

Introduction

Blood pumps or ventricular assist devices (VADs) have only in the past few years changed from a research tool requiring Food and Drug Administration approval for use in a patient to a clinical device available from suppliers. They were born as a spinoff of the work to develop a total artificial heart. Initially, VADs were considered mainly as a research tool to obtain clinical experience with pulsatile blood pumps. Early reports of the use of VADs described their use in desperate clinical scenarios in what were last-ditch efforts to save patients.(1–3) Currently, VADs have a vital role in several aspects of cardiac support. However, complications, including infection, thrombosis, and calcification of the blood contacting surface remain as potential complications of VADs.

Indications for a VAD

Patients who may be considered for VADs can come from varying disease processes that culminate in unilateral or bilateral ventricular failure. Consideration of the physiological reserve of other organ systems is central to patient selection. Most have some degree of renal insufficiency secondary to hypoperfusion. Significant other organ system dysfunction decreases the chances for survival. Use of VADs becomes a surgical judgment of the severity of this dysfunction and the possibility of improvement, with increased cardiac output provided by a VAD. Table 9.1 gives common values considered to indicate ventricular failure, assuming normal ionized Ca^{2+} and the use of maximum inotropic support, which is

Table 8.1

Criteria for Ventricular Failure[a]		
Left Ventricle		*Right Ventricle*
Cardiac Index (L • min^{-1} • m^{-2})	< 1.8	<1.8
Systolic blood pressure (mm Hg)	< 90	See footnote [b]
Mean atrial pressure (mm Hg)	> 20	> 20

[a]*KM, Pae WE, Pierce WS. Circulatory assist devices. In: Hensley FA, Martin DE, eds. A Practical Approach to Cardiac Anesthesia. 2nd ed. Boston: Little, Brown;1995, p500.*

[b]*Right ventricular failure can occur without significant pulmonary hypertension. The work performed by the right ventricle can be inferred from the difference between right atrial and mean pulmonary artery pressures. As this difference approaches zero, flow through the right heart becomes passive, and right ventricular failure is present.*

defined as the use of at least two of the following: >10 µg/kg/min of dopamine; > 10 µg/kg/min of dobutamine; > 0.2 µg/kg/min of epinephrine; > 10 µg/kg/min of amrinone; or > 0.75 µg/kg/min of milrinone. Pennington (4) has also suggested the inclusion of urine output > 20 mL/h and use of an intra-aortic balloon pump as prerequisites for VAD insertion.

Current Assist Pumps

Several blood pumps have been and are being developed for use as ventricular assist devices. The Food and Drug Administration (FDA) overviews medical device clinical trials under the authority given to it by the Food, Drug and Cosmetics Act of 1976. Before a clinical trial begins, the developer must submit to the FDA an application known as an Investigational Device Exemption (IDE). In this application, a complete description is provided of the device, including all materials used in its construction and results of any bench and animal testing as well as a proposal for the clinical trial. The proposal would include patient selection, methods, and an informed consent statement.

Devices that existed before 1976 were not subject to an IDE application. Any new device that can be shown to be "substantially equivalent" to a pre-1976 device can be exempted from the IDE application process by request (510k application). Generally, a 510k application is substantially less expensive and time-consuming than an IDE application. Such devices as balloon pumps and centrifugal pumps are included under this exemption. Once the IDE study is completed, the results are submitted to the FDA for premarket approval (PMA). Only after PMA can a company sell its product.

Abiomed BVS 5000 Biventricular Support System

The Abiomed BVS 5000 device (Abiomed, Inc, Danvers, MA) is a single-use pneumatic pump capable of left, right, or biventricular support (Fig. 8.1). The pump incorporates a dual-chamber design: an atrial (filling) chamber and a ventricular (pumping) chamber, both with a volume of 100 mL. The atrial chamber fills passively from the patient, thus eliminating the need for vacuum, with the attendant risks of air entrainment and atrial collapse. The ventricular chamber alternatively collapses and fills secondary to delivery of compressed air from the console. Each chamber contains a smooth polyurethane bladder. The ventricular chamber is isolated by two polyurethane trileaflet valves to ensure unidirectional flow. The bladders and valves are manufactured from Angioflex, Abiomed's proprietary biomaterial. Cannulation is achieved via the atria using a 46-French, wire-reinforced cannula. The arterial cannula incorporates a 14-mm woven Dacron graft, coated with elastomer to reduce bleeding and eliminate the need for preclotting before implantation. The graft is anastamosed end-to-side to the ascending aorta or pulmonary artery. The cannulas are exteriorized subcostally. A Dacron velour sleeve on the exterior of each cannula promotes tissue ingrowth, which minimizes the risk of infection. The FDA gave premarket approval for the Abiomed Biventricular Support System for the treatment of post-cardiotomy shock in 1992.

The control system monitors the flow of air to and from the blood pumps through the drive line tubing. This provides information on stroke volume (during pump systole) and ventricular bladder filling (during pump diastole), which allows assessment of pump performance. By continuously monitoring air flow, the computer adjusts the duration of pump systole and diastole, pump rate, and pump flow. A closed-loop control algorithm adjusts these parameters to accommodate the flow of blood returning from the patient and to maintain the pump stroke volume near its 80-mL target value. Weaning controls allow each pump to be independently decreased in increments of 0.1 L/min, down to a minimum of 0.5 L/min. If the patient fails to tolerate this reduced pump flow, the weaning mode is turned off, and the pump automatically returns to the full-flow mode.

Hemopump

The Hemopump (Nimbus, Johnson & Johnson, Rancho Cordova, Calif) is an implantable intravascular device that creates non-pulsatile flow. The design is an axial flow pump mounted on a flexible catheter. The pump resides in a 7- x 16-mm cylindrical housing at the proximal end of a 20-cm length of flexible inflow cannula. When inserted in a patient, the pump is located in the descending aorta (Fig. 8.2). Blood is aspirated from the left ventricle and pumped directly into the descending aorta.

ABIOMED BVS 5000 BLOOD PUMP

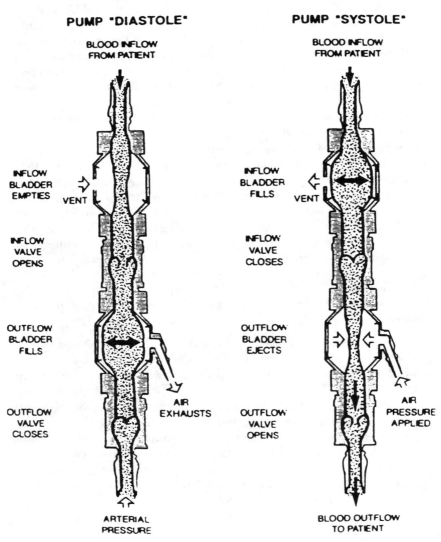

Figure 8.1. *The Abiomed pneumatic assist pump. This is a two-chamber pump, shown in the left panel during diastole and in the right panel during systole. Reprinted with permission from High KM, Pae WE, Pierce WS. Circulatory Assist Devices. In: Hensley FA, Martin DE, eds. A Practical Approach to Cardiac Anesthesia. Boston: Little, Brown; 1995, p 505.*

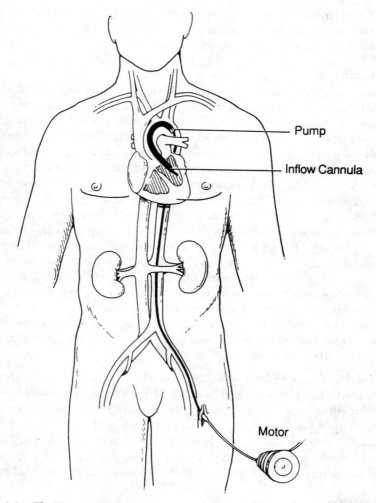

Figure 8.2. *The Hemopump is inserted via one of the femoral arteries. The inflow to the pump sits inside the left ventricle, and the outflow sits in the proximal descending aorta. Reprinted with permission from Arabia FA, Copeland JG, Larson DE, Smith RG, Cleavinger MR. Circulatory assist devices: Applications for ventricular recovery or bridge to transplantation. In: Gravlee GP, Davis RF, Utley JR, eds. Cardiopulmonary Bypass— Principles and Practice. Baltimore: Williams & Wilkins; 1993, p 701.*

The output of the pump is 3 L/min when the pump is rotating at 24,500 rpm, with an afterload of 100 mm Hg.(5) Stationary blades direct the flow as blood exits the pump. The Hemopump is designed for single use and is disposable. Insertion is via the femoral or iliac arteries. This is accomplished through a 12-mm woven graft anastamosed to the artery. The inflow cannula traverses the aortic valve, allowing the distal tip to reside in the left ventricle. Positioning is performed under fluoroscopic guidance. Currently, an IDE is required for use.

Novacor

The Novacor (Novacor Division, Baxter Healthcare Corp, Oakland, Calif) is an implantable, electrically driven left ventricular assist pump. The design uses dual pusher plates to compress a seamless, polyurethane blood sac (Fig. 8.3). The device is encapsulated in a fiberglass-reinforced polymer shell. Electricity is used to energize a solenoid that controls beam springs, which transfer energy from the solenoid to the pusher plates. The blood sac is bonded to the pusher plates. The blood pump volume is 70 mL. The pump can provide flows up to 8 L/min.(6–8) Unidirectional flow is provided by bioprosthetic inflow and outflow valves. Both inflow to and outflow from the pump are carried through low porosity Dacron conduits that traverse the diaphragm. The inflow conduit is attached to a semirigid plastic cannula, which is inserted into a hole cored out of the left ventricular apex. The outflow conduit is usually anastamosed to the ascending aorta; however, it can also be anastamosed to the abdominal aorta. A vent tube from the pump travels subcutaneously and exits the patient in the right lower quadrant of the abdomen. The power and sensor leads from the control panel are contained in the vent tube.

The console contains two controllers; one serves as a backup. Displacement transducers located on the pusher plates and solenoid send information about filling, stroke volume, pump rate, and energy use to the console for display. The Novacor can be triggered to be: (1) at a fixed rate, (2) synchronized to the R wave of the patient's electrocardiogram, or (3) emptying when volume of pump is full. The drive console contains an uninterruptible power supply with 40 minutes of battery backup.

Pierce-Donachy

The Pierce-Donachy pump is a pneumatically driven ventricular assist pump, which can be used to support both the right and left ventricles.(9, 10) The pump consists of a single seamless polyurethane blood sac housed in a rigid polysulfone case (Fig. 8.4). Unidirectional flow is provided by tilting disk prosthetic inflow and outflow valves. The maximum stroke volume is 70 mL. The pump produces pulsatile flow rates of 1.3 to 6.5 L/min. The device is paracorporeal, with the inflow and outflow cannulae traversing the chest wall at the level of the diaphragm. For left ventricular assist, the inflow cannula can be placed either in the left atrium or ventricular apex. The outflow cannula is anastamosed to the ascending aorta. For right ventricular assist, the inflow cannula is inserted into the right atrium. The outflow cannula is anastamosed to the pulmonary artery.

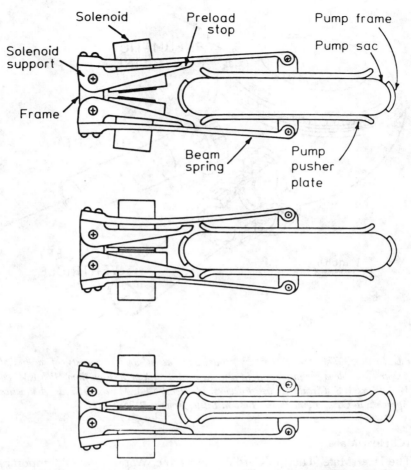

Figure 8.3. *The Novacor pusher plate pump. A metal plate squeezes the bag, which caus-es ejection. The pump is shown in the end-diastolic position (top), at the onset of systole (middle), and in the end-systolic position (bottom). Reprinted with permission from High KM, Pae WE, Pierce WS. Circulatory Assist Devices. In Hensley FA, Martin DE, eds. A Practical Approach to Cardiac Anesthesia. Boston: Little, Brown; 1995, p 506.*

The drive console pressurizes the drive line to cause blood sac emptying and slight negative pressure in pump diastole to promote filling. The Thoratec pump can be triggered: (1) at a fixed rate or (2) in an automatic mode that varies the beat rate to initiate pumping when the blood sac is full. A Hall sensor is used to detect when the pump has filled. The drive console contains an uninterruptible power supply with 40 minutes of bat-tery backup.

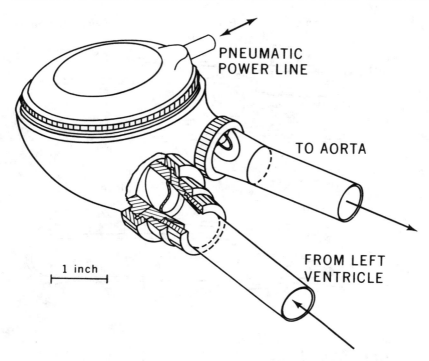

PNEUMATIC
POWER LINE

TO AORTA

FROM LEFT
VENTRICLE

1 inch

Figure 8.4. *The Pierce-Donachy ventricular assist device consists of a flexible polyurethane blood sac inside a rigid case. Reprinted with permission from High KM, Pae WE, Pierce WS. Circulatory assist devices. In: Hensley FA, Martin DE, eds. A Practical Approach to Cardiac Anesthesia. Boston: Little, Brown; 1995, p 505.*

TCI HeartMate

The HeartMate (Thermo Cardiosystems, Inc, Woburn, Mass) temporary pneumatic ventricular assist pump has recently been approved by the FDA as the first assist device to be used as a bridge to heart transplantation. The pump type is a pusher plate with diaphragm (Fig. 8.5). The diaphragm separates the blood chamber from the pusher plate compartment. The outer shell is titanium. The diaphragm is polyurethane bonded to the pusher plate. A mechanical stop determines the maximum full and empty positions of the pusher plate. Maximum volume when full is 218 mL, with a maximum stroke volume of 90 mL. The inlet and outlet valves are 25-mm porcine in a Dacron conduit, housed in a titanium cage. The 19-mm titanium inlet cannula is placed in the left ventricular apex, and the 20-mm woven Dacron graft outlet conduit is anastamosed to the ascending aorta.

The two blood contacting surfaces are one half of the titanium shell and the diaphragm. The titanium surface is textured with sintered titanium

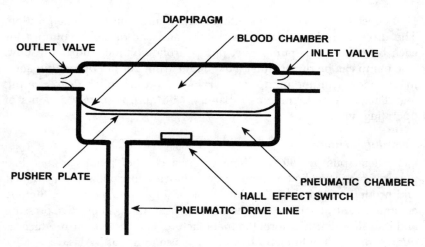

Figure 8.5. *The TCI HeartMate assist pump, which is a pneumatically driven pusher plate pump. Reprinted with permission from High KM, Pae WE, Pierce WS. Circulatory assist devices. In: Hensley FA, Martin DE eds. A Practical Approach to Cardiac Anesthesia. Boston: Little, Brown; 1995, p 506.*

microspheres. The diaphragm surface is textured polyurethane, which under magnification exhibits a microvillous appearance. The initial blood contact with the textured surfaces induces formation of a fibrin-cellular coagulum. Thrombus then forms and is anchored within the interstices of the textured surface by fibrin deposition. Studies have shown this pseudointimal surface to be composed primarily of compact fibrin, types I and II collagen, endothelial cells, and mononucleated cells.(11) Flow cytometry and immunohistochemical staining have demonstrated that pluripotent hematopoietic stem cells colonize the blood surfaces of the pump. Other design elements to minimize areas of stasis and thus the risk of thromboembolic events include a short inflow cannula, a "cornerless" blood chamber, and a wandering flow vortex. The Dacron covered pneumatic drive line promotes fibrous ingrowth, which forms an effective barrier to infection. The pump is placed in a sub-diaphragmatic position in a preperitoneal pocket. Inlet and outlet cannulae traverse the diaphragm. This preperitoneal position minimizes the risks of intraperitoneal adhesions and potential bowel obstruction, which may occur with the pump in an intraperitoneal position. The drive line is tunneled subcutaneously and exits the skin in the left lower quadrant. The TCI HeartMate received PMA in 1994.

The drive system is a portable self-contained unit. It uses a specific volume of room air to cycle the pump. The system is periodically vented to the atmosphere to compensate for any air leakage from the system. A

Hall effect sensor is used to continuously monitor pusher plate position. The drive console displays end-systolic and end-diastolic volumes for each beat as well as pump rate, pump stroke volume, and pump flow. The pump can be run at either a fixed rate (from 20–140 bpm) or in automatic mode, with the pump rate varying according to the degree of filling. The drive unit contains a battery with approximately 2 hours of operating time.

Centrifugal Pumps

Centrifugal pumps will be discussed as a class of pumps rather than pumps from individual manufacturers. They are functionally very similar and produce angular acceleration of blood in a confined space, thereby creating a centrifugal force on the blood, which results in positive pressure and thus flow. Furthermore, the manufacturers promote their products as pumps for cardiopulmonary bypass systems and not as VADs.

Centrifugal pumps have the advantages of availability and ease of use. They are available from multiple manufacturers and have other indications beside ventricular failure. They are used for left atrial-to-aorta bypass for thoracic aortic surgery and sometimes as bypass devices for liver transplantation. This allows the perfusion staff the opportunity to become familiar with the equipment and its operation and warrant the in-house availability of the devices. The individual units also have a compelling cost advantage.

These pumps are relatively easy to use, with the pump output being directly related to both the speed of rotation of the pump and hydrostatic pressure into which it is pumping. Because of the inverse relationship between back pressure and flow, it is necessary to measure the pump flow rate with an electromagnetic flowmeter. Unlike the standard roller pump for cardiopulmonary bypass, it is possible (fortunately) to have the pump spinning at high speeds with a clamp on the inflow cannula without over-pressurization of the tubing and tube rupture. Centrifugal pumps are usually driven and controlled by a reusable drive system, which contains both the electric motor with a rotational speed indicator and the electronics for the electromagnetic flowmeter. There are no centrifugal pumps with PMA for use as VADs. The use here is allowed for compassionate use.

Reports of Use of Assist Pumps

It is difficult to get complete information about the utilization of ventricular assist pumps. A registry for the clinical use of VADs and total artificial hearts (TAHs), which is kept by the American Society of Artificial Internal Organs (ASAIO), tracks blood pump utilization.(12–15) However, reporting is not mandatory, so the registry information provides somewhat limited and incomplete insight into pump use. It appears that there are three major areas of pump use: post-cardiotomy cardiogenic shock (PCCS), bridge to transplantation (bridging), and acute myocardial infarction (AMI). During 1983 to 1993, approximately two thirds of VAD use was for PCCS, approximately 30% for bridging, and only a few percent for AMI. A centrifugal pump was most commonly used (71% of the reported cases) for PCCS, and a pneumatic or electrical motor driven pump was used for bridging to cardiac transplantation (92% of reported cases). However, the reporting of centrifugal pump use has been declining. It is suspected that this represents more a decreased rate of reporting rather than an actual decrease in use. The reported use of the total artificial heart has been declining, and there were no reported uses between 1993 and 1994.

From the ASAIO registry data, it can be seen that the centrifugal pumps were preferentially used for PCCS.

Reports of Complications Common to Prosthetic Pumps

The are no studies comparing any of the VADs in terms of complications or survival rates. The registry keeps a summary of reported complications. In PCCS patients, the registry found the following reported complications: bleeding in 48.3% of patients, low cardiac output in 33.1%, and renal failure in 30.7% of these patients. In those patients receiving an assist device as a bridge to transplantation, bleeding was reported as a problem in 42.5% of patients, infection in 28.5% and renal failure in 22.9%. The reported high bleeding rate in PCCS patients undoubtedly reflected the longer times that these patients spent on cardiopulmonary bypass because of their difficulty in being weaned from bypass.

Bleeding

Bleeding after insertion of VADs is extremely common. The ASAIO registry data shows that bleeding was a reported complication in nearly 50% of VAD insertions in both the PCCS and bridge-to-transplantation groups. Bleeding is problematic not only from its blood volume implications and potential compromise of native ventricular function but also as a medium for infection. Bleeding associated with PCCS is not difficult to understand in the light of protracted cardiopulmonary bypass time. However, bleeding remains a problem even in planned, albeit somewhat urgent, use as a bridge to cardiac transplantation. The use of Dacron cuffs around the atrial cannula has been suggested as a method of decreased bleeding at this site.(16) The use of aprotinin has recently been shown to substantially decrease both postoperative chest tube drainage and blood transfusion requirement.(17)

Infection

The incidence of infections related to the use of VADs is reported to be between 20 and 38% of all patients receiving support.(18–22) In 1992, Pifarre (23) reported similar rates of survival in two groups of transplantation patients: one receiving mechanical support as a bridge to transplantation, and one without mechanical support. The only significant difference in the two groups was the high rate of infection (51.7%) in the mechanical support group. It should be noted that an intra-aortic balloon pump was the most common form (67%) of mechanical support. Based upon similar rates of survival between the two groups, these researchers concluded that mechanical support did not adversely affect outcome in patients awaiting transplantation.

The source of infections in VAD patients may be multifactorial. The presence of large percutaneous tubes provides a pathway for infection. This has been partially addressed by the use of flanges at the skin level (24) to stabilize the drive line and prevent pressure necrosis of the drive line. Dacron velour is cemented around the cannulas at the level of the skin. This allows tissue growth into the substance of the tubing and helps in stabilization of the tube in the tissue. In addition, in vivo studies (25, 26) have suggested that there may be a local effect of polyurethane on neutrophil function when in proximity to the polymer. There was no observable effect on neutrophils from peripheral blood of patients who have VADs. However, a decrease in white blood cell and neutrophil count have been noted in animals implanted with the total artificial heart.(27)

As reported from an ASAIO workshop in 1988, the mediastinum, blood, sputum, and drive lines were the most common sites identified as sites of infection.(19, 26) *Staphylococcus epidermidis, Pseudomonas sp, and Candida sp* were reported as the most common organisms. Reports of use of the various types of pumps appear to show no significant difference in the frequency of infection.

Thrombosis

Thrombosis during VAD implantation occurs as a result of blood contact with the prosthetic surface (28–30) or stagnation of flow within the native ventricle.(31) The ASAIO registry results have indicated an overall incidence of embolic or thrombotic events in 10.3% of all patients undergoing ventricular assistance because of post-cardiotomy cardiogenic shock and in 16.6% of all patients undergoing support as a bridge to transplantation. In some of these patients, thrombus formation has been reported on heparin-coated surfaces of pumps even when systemic heparin has been used.(32) Reports regarding the use of the neo-intimal surface in the TCI assist pump have generally been favorable and without evidence of thrombosis or embolization.(11)

Current prophylaxis for thrombosis consists of heparin to maintain a target partial thromboplastin time of 1 1/2 to 2 times normal. At some point after bleeding has stopped, heparin therapy is replaced with warfarin. In addition, anti-platelet therapy is usually undertaken with either aspirin or dipyridamole.

Unsolved Problems

Volume Compensators

In order to have a totally implantable electric VAD, it is essential to incorporate a volume compensation device. This device would in some manner allow for the flow of gas (or liquid) into and from the gas side of the pump during the pumping cycle to accommodate for the changing volume in this space. There are currently no reliable volume compensators available, although several designs are under investigation. Not compensating for the change in gas volume inside the pump would cause high stresses on the flexible blood contacting surface and loading of the drive motors.

Calcification

Calcium deposition on the blood contacting surface of some of the pulsatile pumps has been an intermittent problem.(33–36) It has not been reported to occur on the pseudo-intimal surface of the HeartMate but has been described with the polyurethane blood sac. The occurrence of calcification is variable and progressive with implantation time. It seems to usually be the most severe in regions of the polyurethane sac that undergo the most severe flexing during operation. Speculation centers on the flexing causing fatigue of the polyurethane and microfractures in the polyurethane, which create a nidus for clot and subsequent calcification, but there are no studies to support this mechanism.

Total Artificial Heart

As mentioned previously, the use of the total artificial heart (TAH) has declined in recent years.(13, 14, 37) The TAH had been used as a bridging device in patients with severe biventricular failure who are awaiting cardiac transplantation. Although used for post-cardiotomy cardiogenic shock patients, the primary use of the TAH has been for a bridging device to cardiac transplantation. This occurred naturally because of the complexity and manpower requirements to implant a TAH and the need for rapid cardiovascular support in the PCCS patient.

The TAH by all developers was a biventricular pump designed to fit into the mediastinal cavity after removal of the patient's heart. Dacron sewing rings allowed attachment of the pumps to native remnants. Initial prototypes were all pneumatically driven with percutaneous drive lines and sensing wires. The drive pressure varies in a similar manner to assist pumps, with a super-systolic pressure compressing the blood sac and a sub-atmospheric pressure drawing blood into the pump. The left- and right-sided pumps work asynchronously. Usually, the left side pumped in a full to empty mode and the right side pumped either in a similar manner or at a constant rate. Direct flow through the right pump could occur in a patient who has low pulmonary artery pressures. More recently, totally implanted electric pumps have been designed and tested in animals.

The reason for the decline in use of the TAH can be seen in the ASAIO registry data. During the 10-year period ending in 1993, the discharge from hospital rates were 68.1% in patients receiving bilateral assist devices and 48.9% in patients receiving TAH. The exact reason for the lower survival rates in the TAH group is probably related to higher rates of infection.

Summary

VADs are a fixed part of the algorithm for treatment of ventricular failure, either after cardiopulmonary bypass or in progressive ventricular failure in the pre-transplantation patient. Centrifugal pumps are most commonly employed for ventricular failure after bypass, and one of a number of pulsatile pumps are usually used to bridge patients to transplantation. Totally implantable VADs for patients who have chronic ventricular failure may be the future for these devices. The total artificial heart seems to have an uncertain future.

REFERENCES

1. Pierce WS. Artificial hearts and blood pumps in the treatment of profound heart failure. Circulation 1983;68:883–888.
2. Norman JC, et al. Total support of the circulation of a patient with post-cardiotomy stone-heart syndrome by a partial artificial heart (ALVAD) for 5 days followed by heart and kidney transplantation. Lancet 1978;1:1125–1127.
3. Berger RL, Merin G, Carr J, Sossman HA, Bernhard WF. Successful use of a left ventricular assist device in cardiogenic shock from massive postoperative myocardial infarction. J Thorac Cardiovasc Surg 1979;78:626–632.
4. Pennington DG, Joyce LD, Pae WE Jr, Burkholder JA. Circulatory support 1988. Patient selection. Ann Thorac Surg 1989;47:77–81.
5. Butler KC, Moise JC, Wampler RK. The Hemopump—A new cardiac prosthesis device. IEEE Trans Biomed Eng 1990;37:193–196.
6. Shinn JA. Novacor left ventricular assist system. AACN Clin Issues Crit Care Nurs 1991;3:575–586.
7. Miyamoto Y, et al. Hemodynamic parameters influencing clinical performance of Novacor left ventricular assist system. Artif Organs 1990;14:454–457.
8. Mandarino WA, et al. Novacor left ventricular assist filling and ejection in the presence of device complications. ASAIO Trans 1990;36:M387–M389.

9. Weiss WJ, et al. A completely implanted left ventricular assist device. Chronic in vivo testing. ASAIO J 1993;39:M427–M432.

10. Davis PK, Pae WE Jr, Pierce WS. Toward an implantable artificial heart. Experimental and clinical experience at The Pennsylvania State University. (Review). Invest Radiol 1989;24:81–87.

11. Graham TR, et al. Neo-intimal development on textured biomaterial surfaces during clinical use of an implantable left ventricular assist device. Eur J Cardiothorac Surg 1990;4:182–190.

12. Pae WE Jr. Ventricular assist devices and total artificial hearts: A combined registry experience. Ann Thorac Surg 1993;55:295–298.

13. Oaks TE, Pae WE Jr, Miller CA, Pierce WS. Combined registry for the clinical use of mechanical ventricular assist pumps and the total artificial heart in conjunction with heart transplantation: Fifth official report–1990. J Heart Lung Transplant 1991;10:621–625.

14. Johnson KE, Liska MB, Joyce LD, Emery RW. Registry report. Use of total artificial hearts: Summary of world experience, 1969–1991. ASAIO J 1992;38:M486–M492.

15. Pae WE Jr, Pierce WS. Combined registry for the clinical use of mechanical ventricular assist pumps and the total artificial heart: first official report–1986. J Heart Transplant 1987;6:68–70.

16. Wyatt DA, Kron IL, Tribble CG. Use of a Dacron cuff to decrease bleeding from atrial cannulas of ventricular assist devices. Ann Thorac Surg 1993;55:1264–1265.

17. Pae WE Jr, Aufiero TX, Weldner PW, Miller CA, Pierce WS. Aprotinin therapy for insertion of ventricular assist devices for staged heart transplantation. J Heart Lung Transplant 1994;13:811–816.

18. Pennington DG, et al. Seven years' experience with the Pierce-Donachy ventricular assist device. J Thorac Cardiovasc Surg 1988;96:901–911.

19. Burns GL. Infections associated with implanted blood pumps. (Review). Int J Artif Organs 1993;16:771–776.

20. Farrar DJ, Hill JD. Univentricular and biventricular Thoratec VAD support as a bridge to transplantation. Ann Thorac Surg 1993;55:276–282.

21. Pennington DG, McBride LR, Miller LW, Swartz MT. Eleven years' experience with the Pierce-Donachy ventricular assist device. J Heart Lung Transplant 1994;13:803–810.

22. Murakami T, et al. Results of circulatory support for postoperative cardiogenic shock. Artif Organs 1994;18:691–697.

23. Pifarre R, et al. Comparison of results after heart transplantation: mechanically supported versus nonsupported patients. J Heart Lung Transplant 1992;11:235–239.

24. Topaz PA, Topaz SR, Kolff WJ. Molded double lumen silicone skin button for drivelines to an artificial heart. ASAIO Trans 1991;37:M222–M223.

25. Kaplan SS, et al. Biomaterial associated impairment of local neutrophil function. ASAIO Trans 1990;36:M172–M175.

26. Didisheim P, et al. Infections and thromboembolism with implantable cardiovascular devices. (Review). ASAIO Trans 1989;35:54–70.

27. Al-Mondhiry H, Pae WE Jr, Rosenberg G, Pierce WS. Hematologic and hemostatic complications associated with long-term use of total artificial heart: clinical and experimental observations. Artif Organs 1992;16:83–89.

28. Christie AM, Donachy JH, Rosenberg G, Pierce WS. Scanning electron microscopic evaluation of polyurethanes used for biomedical applications. ASAIO Trans 1985;31:512–516.

29. Mesana T, Monties JR, Blin D, Goudard A, Mouly-Bandini A, Cornen A. Thromboembolytic complications during circulatory assistance with a centrifugal pump in patients with valvular prostheses. ASAIO Trans 1990;36:M525–M528.

30. Takano H, et al. Multi-institutional studies of the National Cardiovascular Center Ventricular Assist System: Use in 92 patients. ASAIO Trans 1989;35:541–544.

31. Nakatani T, et al. Thrombus in a natural left ventricle during left ventricular assist: Another thromboembolic risk factor. ASAIO Trans 1990;36: M711–M714.

32. Bianchi JJ, et al. Initial clinical experience with centrifugal pumps coated with the Carmeda process. ASAIO J 1992;38:M143–M146.

33. Tomazic BB, Brown WE, Queral LA, Sadovnik M. Physiochemical characterization of cardiovascular calcified deposits. I. Isolation, purification and instrumental analysis. Atherosclerosis 1988;69:5–19.

34. Coleman DL. Mineralization of blood pump bladders. Trans Am Soc Artif Intern Organs 1981;27:708–713.

35. Levy RJ, et al. Cardiovascular implant calcification: A survey and update. (Review). Biomaterials 1991;12:707–714.

36. Pierce WS, Donachy JH, Rosenberg G, Baier RE. Calcification inside artificial hearts: Inhibition by warfarin-sodium. Science 1980;208:601–603.

37. Miller CA, Pae WE Jr, Pierce WS. Combined registry for the clinical use of mechanical ventricular assist pumps and the total artificial heart in conjunction with heart transplantation: Fourth official report–1989. J Heart Transplant 1990;9:453–458.

Index